EPIGENETIC ROADMAP
to
PARENTING CHILDREN
with
ADHD

Manage Challenging Behaviors,
Foster Harmonious Family Relationships,
and Honor Neurodiversity

ALICIA MAZARI-ANDERSEN PHD
AND BRENDA WOLLENBERG

This publication is designed to provide accurate and authoritative information regarding the subject matter covered. It is sold with the understanding that the authors do not render medical services. Please seek a competent professional for medical advice or other expert assistance.

Cover design by Ashish Joshi.

Disclaimer: The authors make no guarantees about the results you will achieve by reading this book. All successful wellness attempts require work. The results and client stories presented in this book represent results achieved working directly with the authors. Your results may vary when undertaking any new wellness journey.

To our brilliant, kind, and loving families, who have patiently endured countless discussions on wellness and epigenetics (with only a modest amount of eye-glazing), and especially to Rachel, who generously and vulnerably allowed us to weave her story throughout the book.

And to Dr. Penny Kendall-Reed, our appreciated and esteemed teacher and mentor in the science and art of gene analysis and interpretation—without your guidance, our work in personalized nutrition and this book would not exist.

Thank you!

Contents

Chapter 1

Introduction

It was the night before the moving truck arrived to take my (Brenda's) family to our new home. Things were a little chaotic, but the "plate juggling" seemed to be going well, that is, until I walked into Rachel's room. Like the other three of our five kids who still were of the age to live at home with my husband, Mark, and me, Rachel (15) had been given a clear set of instructions around her responsibilities in the move. Each of the kids' bedrooms had been stocked with empty boxes, and throughout the previous two weeks, we'd been touching base with them to encourage them to get little bits done each day.

Joel (18) was ready to go, and Bekah (12) was close. However, I walked into Rachel's room to what amounted to a clothing explosion. Most packing boxes were virtually empty, and in the middle of the mayhem, Rachel was sitting on her barely visible bed, reading a book.

Though I managed to keep a reasonably civil tone, let's just say the conversation didn't go well. I was on a high horse of "family members' responsibility to be contributing parts of the household," and not for the first time, I felt a bit of woundedness that it seemed Rachel expected to be bailed out at the last minute by me. But Rachel was simply overwhelmed at the pile of work still to be done (and therefore practicing her go-to procrastination strategy, her love of reading) and frustrated at me ("You already told me all this earlier this week, mom," and "I'll get it done!").

Fast-forward 15 years. Rachel, a kind, intelligent, loving, justice-focused, and funny young woman working as a lawyer, was preparing to move households. I'd offered to come and help her for a few hours on a Saturday morning.

With Rachel being diagnosed with ADHD several years previous, both she and I had a whole different set of understanding and coping mechanisms. I'd also learned much more about epigenetics (the impact of the environment—nurture—on gene expression—nature) and had provided Rachel with a personalized-to-her set of suggestions regarding nutritional intake, supplements, and mindfulness.

In turn, she had tackled counseling, exercise (organizing team sports for her law firm members and outside friends), judicious medication use, and regularly enjoyed creative activities like pottery and watercolor painting.

With those tools, our move experience was like night and day from the one we'd had in Rachel's mid-teens. We tackled one room (her bedroom) and one set of tasks (sorting her clothes). We prepped boxes or bags for "keeping" (summer and winter designations), for "donating" (here is where I scored a few lovely items!), and for "consigning." We talked a lot throughout the morning, checking in to see whether we needed a tea or refueling break.

When I left Rachel's place, after a big hug and multiple "thanks" all around for such a great morning together, I reflected on the differences that proper diagnosis and understanding of neurological diversity can make. I rejoiced that Rachel hadn't simply accepted the labeling and commonly believed outworkings of that diagnosis as something set in stone but that she had worked to highlight her strengths and better manage situations where some of her ADHD traits were a mismatch with successful handling of that situation.

In a nutshell, Rachel's story illustrates a journey of immense possibility.

Epigenetic Roadmap to Parenting Children with ADHD: Manage Challenging Behaviors, Foster Harmonious Family Relationships, and Honor Neurodiversity can guide you and your child, simply and successfully, along that journey.

Our book is about more than managing ADHD through childhood and teen years, however. It is based on the belief that genetic diversity, including typical and neurodiverse brain functioning, contributes to human adaptability and, in fact, to humanity. It is built on the concept that ADHD is about differences rather than deficits and values the many beautiful facets of our ADHD children's personalities and gifts.

Within that frame of reference—valuing neurodiversity while acknowledging the life challenges it presents—we delve into epigenetic factors contributing to ADHD and provide suggestions that could potentially help your child better handle those challenges.

At this point, you might be wondering:

- Who we are, why we wrote this book and who it's for.

- How we hope to guide you to an expanded way of looking at ADHD.

- What new perspectives and insights we can provide that enable parents to see the light in what can sometimes feel like a very long ADHD tunnel.

We are Alicia Mazari-Andersen and Brenda Wollenberg, and we bring a wealth of passion and experience to this journey. We have decades of experience as nutritionists and a nutritional education based on decades of experience in other fields. But before all those years of higher education, and one of the primary reasons we wrote this book, we were sickly kids!

I (Alicia) had digestive issues (think severe constipation due to diet and an ingrained belief that one shouldn't use public bathrooms!) and a range of ADHD-type symptoms. Then, after a move from my birthplace in Mexico, where I completed a Bachelor's and Master's degree in Biology, to Vancouver for my PhD work in Botany, I had issues with hormonal balance and carrying too much body fat for my size of frame.

I (Brenda) suffered from rheumatic fever at five years of age and then moved on to stressful late childhood and teen years that triggered anxious thoughts and insomnia. By my mid-20s, as a newly graduated social worker, along with my hot-off-the-press degree, I had an ulcer, hypothyroidism, and a sugar/ultra-processed food addiction. And, like Alicia, I dealt with severe constipation.

To say that neither of us was a picture of physical or emotional health would be a massive understatement. We'd love to help others escape that scenario or never have to land there!

Thankfully, at 24 years of age, I (Brenda) met and followed the counsel of a holistic health practitioner who got me started on the wellness journey. Later, both Alicia and I trained in nutrition. We changed our lives by adopting the holistic dietary and lifestyle recommendations we covered in our nutrition coursework. Based on what we have learned more recently about epigenetics—the impact of inner and outer environment on gene expression—we realize we accidentally "reset" our genes (more on this phrase to come) to optimal expression.

Now, we love using Alicia's 30 years of science teaching experience in higher education and Brenda's decade of social work supporting clients' efforts to achieve better mental and emotional health, together with technology and understanding that has developed since the mapping of the human genome to interpret metabolic and genetic profiles and create individualized wellness plans. Beyond that interpretation, we're also pretty darn good at helping our clients implement those wellness plans in their daily lives.

How would we like you to consider looking at ADHD?

As mentioned:

1. The "D"s in ADHD should be considered Differences rather than Deficit or Disorder.

2. Recognition that your child brings a set of unique and valuable traits to this world.

However, the book isn't written by authors living in "La La Land." We know that some of the same neurodivergent traits that help children excel and contribute can also foster challenges in situations that better match neurotypical functioning. Therefore, this book contains plenty of insight into tools that help children self-regulate, grow in emotional maturity and executive function, and better handle situations where their typical operating style is at odds with what the situation requires.

In a nutshell, understanding ADHD is about understanding the intricate balance between nature, the genetic information one has been given, and nurture, the physical, emotional, and mental care that can be provided to allow that genetic information to be optimally expressed. This book explores how genetic predispositions interact with environmental factors, allowing you to create a roadmap that supports your child and your family in the most effective and personalized manner possible.

The focus of *Epigenetic Roadmap to Parenting Children with ADHD* is to equip parents and caregivers with strategies grounded in epigenetics to support younger ADHD brains, where executive function continues to develop until around age 25. However, while this book centers on children and teens, the principles of ADHD and epigenetics apply broadly to all ages. Given the genetic nature of ADHD—and that children with ADHD often have at least one parent with the condition—we expect many adults reading this book will find insights and "Aha!" moments for themselves as well. A future volume will specifically explore the role of epigenetics in ADHD in adults.

Our book is structured around seven Core Steps: Eat, Move, Sleep, Detox, Calm, Inflammation and Repair. To make things easier to remember, you can think of the Core Steps as a simple ELEVATE acronym:

- **E** - Eat for Energy

- **L** - Love to Move

- **E** - Enjoy Sleep

- **V** - Value Detox

- **A** - Access Calm

- **T** - Target Inflammation

- **E** - Engage Repair

After our Introduction and ADHD Primer, we will explore each Core Step and wrap up the book with three Supplemental Essentials: Behavioral and Educational Interventions, ADHD Family Dynamics, and Medical and Alternative Treatments.

Throughout this book, we'll combine scientific concepts with relatable anecdotes, simplified examples, and case studies. We aim to create a sturdy, easy-to-navigate bridge between complex ideas and practical applications—one you won't need ten years of study to cross. This approach ensures the information feels understandable and immediately actionable for your family. Our overall hope is that you will elevate the happiness and health of not only your child with ADHD but also you as their parent.

Based on reviews of Brenda's last book, *Metabolic Health Roadmap,* and its design, which made it easy for readers to absorb and implement its suggestions, *Epigenetic Roadmap to Parenting Children with ADHD* will follow a similar format.

We'll give you a **TRAVEL SIZE VERSION SUMMARY** at the start of each Step. Then, we'll have you visit an **INFORMATION CENTER,** where we will "show you the science" while keeping that science as simple as possible.

If our recent six-plus years of work in epigenetics have taught us anything, it is that we are body, mind, and spirit connected. Therefore, we'll follow that science up with some **TRAVELER ASSISTANCE**. These are tools or bits of information to support you in parenting a child with ADHD. They are relevant not simply to a specific Step but to the overall journey, and they often focus on the hidden benefits of having an ADHD brain!

Next, we'll have you take a **REST STOP**. This allows you and your child time to reflect or sit quietly with what you've read. And, because traveling almost always includes some **ROADWORK,** we'll give you and your child a small but helpful activity to complete.

Your child can track their progress on this journey while doing fun activities in the companion *Happy, Healthy Kids Activity Book* (available for free download here: https://www.inbalancelm.com/ADHD_kidsbook-triplog. Parents can also note their reflections on paper, in a digital notebook, or in the complementary parent Trip Log (available for free download at the same link). Do you have an older child with ADHD? Teens can note their reflections wherever they choose or use a copy of the Trip Log.

Finally, what is a road trip without a **SOUVENIR**? At the end of each Step, we will provide a suggested souvenir. These will motivate you and your child on the journey and celebrate the success you have achieved to that point. Our goal is to provide a comprehensive roadmap that you can easily apply in your family's day-to-day life.

Besides the road trip format, what also sets this book apart is its unique focus on the impact of environmental changes on gene expression—the previously mentioned concept known as epigenetics. We don't view ADHD as a deficit but as a different way of experiencing the world. In an adaptation of a social media post I (Brenda) saw recently, we see those with ADHD as normal cheetahs, not malfunctioning tigers.

By recognizing ADHD strengths and addressing ADHD behavioral challenges—situations for which we use the term "mismatches," first encountered in Siddhartha Mukherjee's brilliant book *The Gene: An Intimate History*—we can create environments that support and nurture our children with ADHD. Including epigenetic science offers insights not typically covered in mainstream parenting guides, making this book a valuable resource for any parent navigating the ADHD journey.

We will not pretend to walk in your shoes or completely understand your household's daily demands. Depending on, among other factors, your child's dopamine metabolism and the activity of their dopamine receptors, you may be dealing with angry outbursts, challenges in the educational system, and a child who alternates between being kind, gentle, and funny and aggressively mean and volatile.

You know your child far better than we ever will and likely have already gathered a toolkit of strategies that often work for your child—a toolkit that perhaps includes some of the strategies we will present here.

However, our understanding of epigenetics, as it relates to ADHD, means we can offer you additional insight and tools that may fundamentally change how you approach ADHD and partner with your child to help them experience as fulfilling and harmonious a life as possible.

As a parent of a child diagnosed with ADHD as a young adult (Brenda) and someone who experiences many ADHD symptoms (Alicia), we can, however, imagine some of the challenges you face and are here to offer not just hope but concrete strategies. We acknowledge your struggles and assure you the information found here will provide valuable guidance and support.

While this book is not a magic bullet, our commitment to you is to:

- Focus on strengths rather than "deficits."

- Offer actionable solutions rather than unsatisfactory coping mechanisms.

- Support your child's unique epigenetic needs through solid, science-informed data.

- Guide you toward understanding, acceptance, and proactive responsiveness to ADHD symptoms.

- Honor neurodiversity and believe in every individual's potential.

I (Brenda) recently came across a meditative reading on mentorship by Richard Rohr, a Franciscan friar and ecumenical teacher. It discussed not simply telling others how to "fix" their problems so they can be "normal" again. Instead, Rohr relayed that a "true mentor guides people *into* their problems and *through* them."

That is what we aim to do.

Parenting a child with ADHD can feel like an enormous and weighty challenge. We don't want to skirt around complex issues an ADHD brain deals with and how, at times, that brain functioning can create significant mismatches with a situation. We believe that going there—guiding you to understand the contributing factors to ADHD symptoms more thoroughly—and then providing options to walk through those challenges is the best way forward for you and your child.

As Rohr summarized in the mentoring article, "It feels a bit messy and wild, but also wonderful in some way."

We invite you to actively engage with this book, even if it sometimes feels a bit messy and wild.

Gene Expression

OK, we're only a few pages in, and we've already mentioned "gene expression" several times. Let's take a moment to explain it, especially if you have a nagging sense that you kind of know what it means but aren't entirely sure. To do that, we'll use a couple of metaphors.

Gene Expression For Cooks and Music Lovers

Gene expression refers to how the body uses a gene's "instructions" to create proteins that carry out various tasks, such as building structures (e.g., muscle) or triggering actions (e.g., releasing hormones). This process can be compared to following a recipe: the gene is the recipe, and the protein is the finished dish.

However, following this "recipe" can vary depending on factors like environment, stress, diet, or exercise. These factors, which we can influence, can speed up or slow down the execution of the recipe—or even whether it's used.

Instead of sticking with a recipe analogy, and because we love music (in fact, I, Brenda, was listening to my "Gratitude" playlist while writing this section), let's use music to illustrate how genes work and adapt.

Imagine your genes as musicians in an orchestra, each contributing a unique sound or function to your body. Some genes play "softer" notes (quieter expression), while others play "louder" notes (stronger expression). These differences are like each musician's natural tone. Just as a loud trumpet isn't inherently bad, nor is a quiet violin inherently good, genes are not inherently good or bad. Their value depends on the piece being performed and the environment in which they're playing.

The environment acts as the conductor, guiding how the orchestra plays (i.e., modulating gene expression). A booming drumroll might add excitement to a concert hall's triumphant crescendo, but it wouldn't work well during your baby sister's nap. Similarly, a gene coding for impulsivity might spark creativity and quick decision-making in high-energy settings but pose challenges in a classroom that demands focus and quiet.

When the conductor—your environment—is stressed, nutritionally depleted, inflamed, or tired, some orchestra sections may play too loudly (overexpression), while others miss their cues entirely (underexpression). By understanding the "score" of life's demands (e.g., am I at the playground with lots of room to be loud and physically active, is this a time for doing "bunny" breaths so I can come to calm and quiet), the conductor can guide the orchestra to adjust its dynamics, ensuring all instruments—quiet or loud—work together harmoniously.

This is where epigenetics comes in: the conductor's subtle influence over how loudly or softly each musician plays, ensuring the music fits the moment and supports your body's needs.

For other key concepts that may be unfamiliar, see the Glossary of Terms after the book's Conclusion.

Of final note (sorry, we couldn't resist a musical reference), you'll see us repeatedly emphasize the role of inflammation and stress in gene expression—and there's a compelling reason why.

As Dr. Penny Kendall-Reed, one of our primary epigenetic educators and mentors, highlights in her books and coursework, inflammation and stress are critical factors in health because they can significantly alter gene expression, effectively causing up to 90% of genes to behave as if they are not functioning properly (i.e., off tune). This happens because inflammation activates stress pathways, disrupting normal gene regulation. These disruptions can impair neurotransmitter function, immune response, and energy metabolism—key systems for managing ADHD symptoms.

Similarly, stress can trigger challenging types of gene expression by increasing cortisol production. Elevated cortisol levels interfere with cellular function and gene regulation, further disrupting critical processes such as neurotransmitter balance, immune function, and metabolic regulation.

Throughout this book, we'll unpack these effects and processes in greater detail. From the outset, though, we want you to understand why managing your and your child's inflammation and stress is vital and why we are so committed to providing the steps and tools to help you do so effectively.

Whew. A beginning explanation of gene expression and the innate value of your child's genes covered; are you ready to start? Let this journey of exploration, understanding, and growing together begin.

Chapter 2

ADHD Primer – Decoding the Basics

"Our genomes are not just codes written into our DNA; they are historical documents ... they respond constantly to the environment, shaping and reshaping who we are."

- Siddhartha Mukherjee, author of The Gene: An Intimate History

S UMMARY - Travel Size Version

Right out of the gate, we'll start our Primer with a letter to you, a parent or caregiver of a child with ADHD. Why is that? While parenting a child with ADHD has some unique, beautiful, and joyous benefits, it can also be hard—very hard.

We would like you to feel seen, encouraged, and infused with at least a spark of hope that things can be good.

Next, the Primer covers a lot of introductory material, so we've broken it down into the following two chapters. In them, you'll discover the following.

The Scientific Framework for Supporting Your Child with ADHD

Understanding ADHD Foundations asks you to think back to when your child was first diagnosed with ADHD, maybe even WAY back to the last time you took a biology course. But don't worry; we'll keep things simple and actionable, breaking complex concepts into manageable steps.

A Recap of ADHD, Diagnostic Rates, and Its Nuances

ADHD stands for Attention Deficit Hyperactivity Disorder, but we prefer to focus on "Difference" rather than "Deficit or Disorder." It's a neurodevelopmental difference shaped by genetics and environment, not poor parenting (though parenting style can play a role), and its diagnostic rates have risen significantly since the condition was first formally recognized. Understanding the convergence of genetics and the environment is critical to understanding why so many children are currently being diagnosed with ADHD and appreciating your child's unique strengths and challenges.

An Integrative Approach to ADHD

Our approach involves assembling a diverse team of healthcare professionals to create a comprehensive treatment plan. You, the parent, take the lead. We'll guide you in building that team and preparing for appointments.

Brain Anatomy and Neurotransmitter Overview

Key brain areas, such as the prefrontal cortex and basal ganglia, and neurotransmitters, such as dopamine, norepinephrine, epinephrine, and serotonin, play crucial roles in ADHD. We'll discuss how these factors influence ADHD and why targeted treatments can help.

Epigenetic Primer

ADHD is polygenic, meaning multiple genes contribute to its development. Environmental factors like diet, exercise, and sleep can influence how these genes express themselves—a concept called epigenetics. The beauty of epigenetics means your child's lifestyle can significantly impact their ADHD symptoms, which puts a lot of control (and responsibility) in your hands!

A Little Biology Lesson

To better understand epigenetics, we'll provide a brief biology lesson to clarify how these processes work.

ADHD Strengths

It's crucial to recognize the strengths of children with ADHD, which often include creativity, enthusiasm, and problem-solving skills. We'll offer tools to help you identify and nurture these gifts.

ADHD Longer Term

ADHD doesn't end with childhood—it has implications throughout adolescence and adulthood. We'll explore what this means for your child as they grow.

Environment and ADHD

Here, we'll dive into the role of the environment in shaping ADHD symptoms. Some experts, like Dr. Gabor Maté, believe environmental factors play a significant role, while others, like Dr. Russell Barkley, emphasize genetics. We'll explore both perspectives and share our thoughts.

Diagnosing ADHD

Diagnosing ADHD is complex and varies by age. We'll direct you to the appendix, listing the diagnostic criteria for children and those over 17.

O.K. Tea or coffee in hand? Let's get started.

INFORMATION CENTER

A Letter (coming with love) for Parents Navigating ADHD

Dear parent:

In the book's introduction, we mentioned that raising a child, particularly a child with ADHD, can be messy. Our goal was to give you lots of ideas for making that journey a little less messy.

However, as one of our book editors—a single mom with ADHD raising a child with ADHD—so astutely and graciously pointed out, we offer a *wide range* of suggested interventions. Each will require time and energy to implement, which are often in short supply when parenting. A number of the suggestions, particularly supplements, require sufficient finances. Additionally, many of them require the uncertain cooperation of a child!

Depending on how long you have been parenting a child with ADHD, the box of tools you already have at your disposal will range from small to large. Some of our suggestions will be easier to use to expand an existing toolbox than they will for a parent who just learned that they need a new one.

Then, factor in genetics (not every child's foundational reasons for ADHD symptoms are the same) and family dynamics (each one will have more or less parental involvement, family or community support, and an inherent starting level of physical and emotional resources) and you begin to understand why each of these interventions will work for some families and children and not for others. And even when they work—which can often take time—they may work sometimes and not others, often with no indication of why that may be. That is not a failure. That is part of the parenting process. (Believe us, we know!).

Finally, factor in the reality that many parents of children with ADHD have ADHD themselves, and the task of implementing strategies that require focus, persistence, and resilience—even helpful ones—can feel overwhelming. It's essential, therefore, to approach these recommendations with flexibility and self-compassion.

Those are a lot of moving pieces! We assembled this information collection about genetics and environmental influences, parenting, and ADHD in general over decades of parenting and education. For the love of all there is, do not try to implement everything in a month. In fact, do not try to implement everything (full stop).

Small steps, over time, lead to the most lasting change. Start with what feels doable or even easy for your family, and build from there (Or don't! If you find one thing that works and stick with it, that's success.). If a particular suggestion doesn't work, well done for discovering that valuable information. We didn't write this book so that you could add 150 recommendations to your life. We wrote it so you could find the best tools for your child and your circumstances.

We (the collective, which includes the authors and said editor) would like to encourage you that every time one or two of the interventions are used (even when they appear not to succeed) and every time you model (even if you model imperfectly and your child does not seem to replicate it), patterns are introduced and reinforced. We believe that even if you can only implement one or two suggestions, they will bear fruit over time and potentially impact your child for the rest of their life.

We also know that structures, routines, motivation, and follow-through can be a challenge for parents with ADHD and that repeated failure to do the things they say are important for themselves and their child can, despite success in other areas, lead to a certain level of resignation and hopelessness.

Whether you have ADHD or not, know we understand that parenting a child with ADHD is never going to be easy. If you find yourself in that spot of overwhelm, here is a set of rules to adopt when interacting with the recommendations in this book:

1. **Choose One Step**: Focus on one Core Step and one or two small changes you want to try. Pick one that seems easy or, at the very least, doable. Give it time before adding more.

2. **Make it a Routine**: Create simple, repeatable routines with that one step; outsource the decision-making, task initiation, and all the other executive functions required for getting things done to a structure of consistency.

3. **Be Kind to Yourself**: Remember that progress is progress, no matter how small. You are here for the long haul, so celebrate wins, even incremental ones.

After carving these three rules in stone, your bonus rule is, when possible, to:

Involve Your Child: Strategize a way to engage your child in a collaborative effort. This isn't always possible, but whenever you can get "buy-in," it helps.

Above all, this book is here to support you, not add to your stress. Use it as a resource to empower your family, but always prioritize your well-being alongside your child's. After all, even when the only recommendation available to you is the solo parent activities that support your health and well-being, as you have a child who is not yet able or willing to participate, you are still making great strides. Truly, a regulated parent is a child's best advocate and guide.

Kind, kind regards,

Alicia and Brenda

PS In some ways, we have unabashedly brought every scrap of good ADHD knowledge we've accumulated over the past four decades to reside on these pages. Sorry. To simplify things, we compiled a "wellness steps for 'those' days" list of suggestions that can be implemented when time, energy, and financial constraints dictate. They are also helpful for any child's DNA. If that resonates, start at the cost-effective Quick Wellness Steps Appendix!

Attention Deficit Hyperactivity Disorder - What's in a Name?

ADHD stands for Attention Deficit Hyperactivity Disorder. It's not a name we're particularly fond of, as it often leads to misconceptions like laziness, lack of intelligence, or even mental illness. "Attention deficit" and "hyperactivity" were initially chosen to describe symptoms like difficulty focusing or sitting still. However, as our understanding of the brain has evolved, we've realized these terms don't fully capture the physiological or emotional realities of ADHD.

Take "deficit," for example. It suggests a shortage, yet many experts now view ADHD as a difference in brain function rather than a deficit. The term "disorder" implies something is fundamentally wrong, but neuroscience has shown these differences are often situational mismatches—where an ADHD brain doesn't align with a specific environment. Imagine a cheetah in a streak of tigers (yes, that's what a group of tigers is called ... who knew!). The cheetah is no less extraordinary than the tiger; it simply thrives under different circumstances.

For this book, while ADHD remains the official term per the DSM-5 (the diagnostic manual for mental health conditions), we prefer to reinterpret the "D" to stand for "Difference" instead of "Deficit." Per our analogy, think of a sleek, fast cheetah versus a strong, powerful tiger. This shift in perspective is vital to honoring the unique ways ADHD brains work while providing tools to manage situations where behavior and environment collide.

Since ADHD-type behavior was first described, it has gone by several names, such as "mental restlessness," "defect of moral control," "hyperkinetic reaction of childhood," and "minimal brain dysfunction." While these terms eventually led to today's ADHD diagnosis, they often carried stigma. Currently, we understand ADHD as a lifelong neurodevelopmental difference influenced by both genetics and environment—not, as sometimes thought, the result of poor parenting.

In this book, we explore the genes that science has linked to ADHD traits and symptoms—the same ones that often give ADHD brains the most grief. These discoveries give us a pathway to reducing those symptoms while reinforcing a vital truth: ADHD is not about something being "wrong" with your child.

Our goal is to help children with ADHD—and their families—see the value and uniqueness they bring to the world. Imagine leaving your child with a safe place to stand, where they're met not with misunderstanding or judgment but with full inclusion and value. Here, they can learn who they are, why they are that way, and how incredible it is to be them. This understanding is a gift not only for your child but also for you as their parent or caregiver.

ADHD doesn't mean your child isn't enough. It means their brain is wired differently, with unique strengths and opportunities. With the right tools, support, and perspective, your family can help them thrive in ways that honor who they indeed are.

ADHD Diagnosis Rates

In the United States, the CDC reports that ADHD prevalence among children aged 4–17 increased from 7.8% in 2003 to 11% in 2011–2012, with current rates stabilizing around 10–11%. Globally, though diagnostic practices vary, ADHD prevalence is estimated at 5–7%. This rise can be attributed in part to expanded diagnostic criteria, improved screening, and greater awareness, particularly regarding ADHD presentations in girls.

Increased public education, advocacy, healthcare provider training, and media coverage have reduced stigma and made parents more likely to seek diagnoses. Beyond these factors, three additional contributors are worth noting: shifts in educational practices, societal emphasis on executive functioning skills (e.g., focus, self-regulation), and environmental factors like increased exposure to toxins or dietary changes.

While we won't cover the first two factors to any degree, note that educational systems have evolved from the more flexible approaches of the past to standardized, structured settings that often favor neurotypical behaviors. This transition has made it harder for neurodivergent children, including those with ADHD, to thrive in environments requiring sustained focus, limited physical activity, and prolonged sitting. Similarly, modern societal values increasingly prioritize executive functioning, further highlighting the challenges faced by individuals with ADHD.

We will, however, cover the profound influence of environmental factors on gene expression in depth (indeed, for the rest of the book!). Specifically, we'll explore how your child's unique genetic makeup interacts with their environment to shape emotional and physical behavior and how you can create a supportive framework for them to flourish.

What ADHD Looks Like

ADHD shows up in different ways. Some children are predominantly inattentive, struggling to focus and often appearing dreamy, while others are hyperactive-impulsive, always moving and acting without thinking. Many have a combination of these traits, making ADHD highly individualized.

In *Healing ADD*, Dr. Daniel Amen, a brain imaging specialist, describes ADHD as an umbrella term covering seven subtypes, with other experts identifying even more variations. Dr. Robert Melillo, a specialist in childhood neurological disorders and author of *Disconnected Kids*, emphasizes hemispheric imbalance, where one side of the brain is underdeveloped compared to the other. He believes this imbalance can affect sensory processing, motor skills, behavior, and social interactions.

This range of different practitioners' theories and approaches can make understanding ADHD feel overwhelming. Instead of getting caught up in labels, however, we suggest you take a step back and think about what ADHD looks like for your child.

Living with ADHD affects daily life in many ways. Children may struggle to stay on task at school, follow instructions, or complete assignments. Routines like getting ready for school or bedtime can become daily battles. Socially, children with ADHD may find it hard to make and keep friends, as impulsive behavior often leads to misunderstandings, aggressive behaviors, or conflicts. And let's not forget procrastination—frequently mistaken for laziness but very different.

Rachel's twas-the-night-before-moving-day story is one small example of these daily struggles (and one that didn't even include perturbed facial gestures, yelling, tears, or phone throws). Yet, these challenges can become manageable with the proper understanding and tools. Various epigenetic changes (e.g., nutrition, supplements, calming practices, medication) can better support neurological functioning, and other environmental changes (e.g., routines, household organization, and focusing on your child's strengths) can alter a situation. Hence, it is more of a "match" with how your child's brain works.

The Integrative Approach to ADHD

An integrative approach is vital for fostering wellness in children with ADHD, encompassing two key aspects:

Collaboration Among Healthcare Practitioners

Consulting with therapists, psychologists, nutritionists, naturopathic doctors, psychiatrists, and pediatricians, each with a unique perspective can provide parents with a range of wellness suggestions.

Ideally, healthcare providers would communicate with each other to create a comprehensive plan for your child. Sadly, this is not the usual reality. Ultimately, your "gut" sense often knows what is best for your child, so remaining in the team lead position usually makes the most sense, interacting with health professionals and ensuring crucial information is shared.

Your child is not just a body, mind, or emotion; they are whole. This integrative approach—both between practitioners and in recognition of your child's whole self—acknowledges the different aspects of your child's makeup.

Epigenetics as an Integrative Lens

Understanding ADHD through an epigenetic lens underscores the interconnectedness of your child's biology and environment. While this book discusses genes across seven distinct categories (Eat, Sleep, Move, Calm, Detox, Inflammation, and Repair), it's crucial to recognize that these genes do not operate in isolation.

For instance, metabolism-related genes are influenced by the foods we eat and the toxic load those foods may introduce. Likewise, sleep genes are affected by stress, creating a bi-directional relationship in which poor sleep exacerbates stress and impairs sleep quality, onset, and duration. Reduced sleep cycles, in turn, diminish the body's ability to detoxify and repair itself overnight.

An integrative approach to epigenetics helps you see these connections and gives guidance on making lifestyle changes that positively influence your child's genetic expression. By considering how various factors—nutrition, stress management, physical activity, and sleep—interact, you can create a comprehensive plan to support your child's ADHD journey and overall wellness.

Brain Anatomy and ADHD

Although we are not neurologists or, in fact, brain specialists of any type, we would like to provide a brief explanation, within our scope of practice, of some brain structures linked to ADHD.

First, note that many regions of the brain have the potential to be involved with ADHD. Depending upon genetics and factors such as injury or stress, your child may exhibit symptoms related to dysregulation in one or more regions.

This dysregulation has the potential to foster delayed executive functioning, a term often linked with ADHD and one that, in many ways, is crucial to both understanding ADHD and informing the best way to respond to children with ADHD.

Expanding on that concept, children with ADHD often experience delays in executive functioning—skills like impulse control, emotional regulation, and flexible thinking can lag behind their peers for several years. For example:

- A 10-year-old with ADHD might react to frustration with yelling or hitting, behaviors more typical of a 6-year-old.

- A 17-year-old may be expected to independently organize, manage, and complete complex homework assignments. However, their ability to initiate tasks and sustain focus might resemble that of a neurotypical 14-year-old.

- Even a simple "no" can feel overwhelming at any age as their brain struggles to evaluate alternative solutions or regulate emotions.

It's important to remember that not all children with ADHD experience these challenges in the same way. However, understanding this tendency can shift a parent's mindset from frustration to empathy when behaviors escalate.

The following chart, taken from Dr. Melillo's work, provides a snapshot of eight key brain regions, some of which are integral to executive functioning, that could impact your child's ADHD symptoms.

Key Regions in the Brain Involved in ADHD

PREFRONTAL CORTEX (PFC)	BASAL GANGLIA	CORPUS CALLOSUM	CEREBELLUM
In ADHD, the PFC often shows reduced activity and connectivity, leading to difficulties with focusing, organizing tasks, controlling impulses, and regulating behavior.	Individuals with ADHD often have structural and functional abnormalities in the basal ganglia, which may result in hyperactivity, motor control issues, and problems with processing rewards, contributing to impulsive behavior.	Reduced size or structural differences in ADHD may impair interhemispheric communication, affecting coordination of attention, emotion regulation, and cognitive tasks.	It is often smaller or functions differently in people with ADHD, contributing to motor coordination issues, poor timing, and difficulties with sustained attention.
HIPPOCAMPUS	**AMYGDALA**	**THALAMUS**	**BRAINSTEM**
Dysfunction can contribute to difficulties with memory, learning, and processing new information, which are common symptoms in ADHD.	Alterations in ADHD may lead to emotional impulsivity, difficulties with emotional regulation, and increased sensitivity to stress.	Abnormalities may affect sensory processing, alertness, and the ability to filter out irrelevant information, contributing to inattention and distractibility.	Dysfunction may affect arousal, sleep patterns, and autonomic regulation, which can exacerbate symptoms such as inattention, hyperactivity, and impulsivity.

Dr. Robert Melillo 2024

Note, too, that the Core Steps we cover in this book can impact brain function independently of brain region size or structure. Let's look, for example, at the prefrontal cortex (PFC)—a region responsible for executive function and linked to ADHD. Environmental factors like inflammation and stress can lead to PFC underactivity, redirecting dopamine to other brain regions. This shift often results in impulsivity, attention loss, poor decision-making, and the familiar exclamation, "I want it now!"

While the PFC doesn't directly produce dopamine, it relies on finely tuned regulation of dopamine to function optimally. The importance of the PFC's activity has led to most of the research on ADHD medications addressing dopamine balance.

Understanding the crucial role dopamine plays in motivation and reward and the inherent drive your child with ADHD will have to seek out behaviors and activities that stimulate dopamine is a vital foundation in wellness planning for your child. We'll dive deeper into dopamine pathways in the Calm Step and Medical and Alternative Treatment Supplementary Essentials. While we'll keep the main discussion about inflammation to Step Six – Inflammation, you will start to read about its effects and ways to address it from the beginning in Step One – Eat.

Stress and Neurotransmitters in ADHD

For our purposes, it is essential to understand that neurotransmitters like dopamine, norepinephrine, and serotonin play a critical role in brain functioning in general, specifically with ADHD. For a detailed discussion of the mechanics of these interactions, we recommend reading sources that are scientifically credible yet easy to understand (e.g., *The Molecule of More* by Daniel Z. Lieberman, MD, and the TED Talk by Stephen Tonti, ADHD As a Difference in Cognition, Not a Disorder).

For now, however, recognize that chemicals like dopamine, norepinephrine, and serotonin play a critical role in ADHD by regulating attention, impulsivity, mood, and hyperactivity. Dopamine is the brain's "feel-good" messenger, crucial for motivation and reward. Low dopamine or a lack of receptors can lead to procrastination, impulsivity, and poor time management symptoms that I (Alicia) can tell you are very real. There are days when procrastination takes over my being, and time management can be challenging!

However, seeking to elevate low dopamine levels can manifest in even more challenging ways, such as substance abuse, self-harm, and high-risk behaviors.

Norepinephrine helps with alertness and focus, while serotonin regulates mood. Imbalances in these neurotransmitters can make it hard for your child to stay on task and may contribute to emotional ups and downs.

As mentioned with brain region size and structure, keep in mind that more than just neurotransmitter levels may be at play—diet, inflammation, stress, and sleep can also affect brain activity. When these brain regions are out of sync, it shows up as difficulty focusing, forgetting tasks, or acting impulsively. Understanding these brain dynamics helps explain why structured routines and behavioral therapy can be so effective.

These neurological insights also have practical implications for treatment. Medications like stimulants boost dopamine and norepinephrine levels, improving focus and reducing impulsivity. Behavioral interventions, such as cognitive therapy, can help your child develop strategies to manage their symptoms effectively.

We'll draw on insights from professionals like Dr. Amen, Dr. Melillo, and Dr. James Greenblatt, a holistic psychiatrist, to show how targeted treatments and lifestyle changes—such as personalized diets, circadian rhythm support, regular exercise, and possibly resetting (i.e., positively modulating) the Hypothalamic-Pituitary-Adrenal axis (more of this in Step Five – Calm)—form a holistic strategy for managing ADHD.

DNA Primer and Perspectives: How DNA Influences ADHD

First, note that ADHD is a polygenic rather than a monogenic condition. That means the many symptoms included in an ADHD diagnosis do not come from a single gene (monogenic) but instead can arise from a wide range of genes (polygenic). And those symptoms will not be fostered by the same gene coding amongst all children diagnosed with ADHD. This is where we truly begin to see the impact of personalized nurture (i.e., environment) on nature (i.e., genetics). To better understand the differences between monogenic and polygenic diseases, read Siddhartha Mukherjee's book *The Gene: An Intimate History*. Among many other outstanding gene topics, it explains these concepts excellently.

The fact that many genes influence ADHD types of expression means a vast number of genes could be included in our book. While we do indeed cover a lot of genes, the number could have been much higher.

So, which genes made the cut, and why? We ran possible genes through our 3-R Rating system to determine which to include in our material. Then, we added a fourth "R" for you, as a parent, to use as a filter in determining which suggestions to consider.

Scientific Research - We look at genes with credible scientific literature backing their link to ADHD, including scientific references for animal and human studies.

Clinical Relevance - Just because a gene and its variant have a relatively large amount of scientific research, however, does not ensure its inclusion in our book. The results of that research needed to demonstrate clinical relevance to ADHD or other relevant conditions (e.g., inflammation, cortisol dysregulation) that could potentially foster ADHD symptoms. We learned through training and mentoring with Dr. Penny Kendall-Reed ND, a specialist in the analysis and interpretation of genetic profiles, that the most beneficial results occur when we work with Single Nucleotide Polymorphisms (SNPs: genetic variations that we'll expand on shortly!) that respond to environmental changes and have years of clinical research. For our evaluation of clinically relevant genes, we appreciate the clinical studies shared by Dr. Kendall-Reed, which showed her more than 20 years of work with patients in Ontario, Canada.

Responsiveness to Environmental Changes - Even a gene with solid scientific research and clinical relevance to ADHD needed to meet a third criterion to be included. The gene had to be responsive to environmental change. Therefore, in either the body of research or case studies of children with whom we are familiar, someone who made the epigenetic changes mentioned in our book must have achieved positive results.

Personal Relevance - This point relates to the fact that if the gene is not relevant to your child's personal ADHD history (i.e., there are no signs this gene is playing a role in your child's symptoms), it may be a gene to which you do not need to pay attention.

Gene 4-R Rating

SCIENTIFIC RESEARCH	CLINICAL RELEVANCE	RESPONSIVE TO ENVIRONMENTAL CHANGES	PERSONAL RELEVANCE
Genes that have been researched both in animal and human studies. Grounded in science.	Backed up by over 20 years of clinical studies done by Dr. Penny Kendall-Reed.	Environmental factors, such as food and supplements, can change the expression of these SNPs.	Genes that are relevant to your child's personal ADHD history.

In addition to this critical way of understanding why the SNPs we work with are relevant, it is essential to point out that people often only look at "end" genes. For example, do I have the Alzheimer's gene or the breast cancer gene ... the type of genes that create a propensity for someone to develop a disease? These are end rather than "trigger" genes, a concept we learned from Dr. Kendall-Reed. To understand the difference, we'll give you an analogy.

What do you need to start a bonfire? Usually, it is small branches, kindling, matches, or some paper. When the fire starts, you might throw in bigger dried logs so it burns hotter and lasts longer. Imagine that the roaring fire is those end genes.

But what did that fire need to get it going? It required trigger genes. Trigger genes are the kindling, paper, and matches at the beginning of the process. And so, if inflammation, for example, is a bonfire, how do you turn it off? Direct your attention to what was needed to start the inflammation fire, such as the trigger genes like metabolic genes (e.g., eating an anti-inflammatory diet) or detoxification genes (e.g., minimizing household toxins and supporting liver functioning).

If you understand how to ensure those trigger genes are working optimally—something Dr. Kendall-Reed calls the "Goldilocks" position—then there will likely not be a bonfire (i.e., end genes turning on).

In our online searches, we usually encounter research focusing on end genes. However, in most instances, it is best to start small and catch the fire when it is manageable (i.e., where addressing trigger genes could keep that fire more manageable) rather than allowing it to burn at full blast and become a forest fire.

A Short Biology Lesson

Now that you understand our gene selection process for the book, let's consider a mosaic analogy. Imagine the body as an enormous and beautiful collection of mosaic tiles. Imagine these tiles as instructions for what each piece makes to build and maintain your cells. These tiles are your DNA, the blueprint for everything about you. Genes are like colors on that tile, instructing your body to build and maintain itself.

DNA is housed in the nucleus of each cell, and it's made up of nucleotides, which are the basic building blocks of nucleic acids. A nucleotide consists of a sugar molecule (deoxyribose for DNA) attached to a phosphate group and a nitrogen-containing base. The bases found in a DNA molecule are Adenine (A), Guanine (G), Cytosine (C), and Thymine (T).

These bases pair up to form the rungs of the DNA ladder, creating a unique genetic code for every individual. This code is what makes you, you. Each gene contains a specific sequence that "codes for" the production of a protein. In other words, the gene provides instructions that guide the cell in making a particular protein, which could serve various functions within the cell (e.g., acting as an enzyme, transporter, receptor, etc.). That protein, in turn, supplies the information cells need to differentiate, reproduce, and grow.

Within each pair of bases we get from our parents, we can receive either normal single nucleotide polymorphisms (also called wild-type base SNPs, as they are found most commonly in the wild) or variant SNPs.

Single nucleotide polymorphisms (SNPs) occur normally in a person's DNA. Each SNP represents a genetic variation within a single DNA building block in a gene sequence. Imagine these SNPs or variations as changes in one letter within your DNA, almost like a "typo." It doesn't mean that your genes are not doing their job, necessarily (i.e., producing proteins), but that they may have a reduced capacity to express themselves or send different messages.

Being *variant* or *normal*—terms that describe the frequency of a specific gene coding in the population rather than indicating one as inherently better—can influence how you respond to particular scenarios. For instance, you might be more or less likely to trigger gut inflammation in response to carbohydrate intake, or you could have a genetic predisposition to remain in a fight-or-flight state under stress. These genetic differences shape your unique biological reactions.

To make the concept easier to understand, we've developed a "coloring system" in which normal SNPs are represented as green, heterozygous SNPs as yellow, and variant SNPs as red. This color coding is not intended to suggest the moral superiority of one coding over another but instead serves as a guide, much like a traffic light.

- **Green coding (normal SNPs)** generally suggests optimal functionality or a trait that provides a benefit in most situations. Thus, we can "sail through the green light" with little need for intervention other than continuing to support that helpful gene expression.

- **Yellow coding (heterozygous SNPs)** signals a potential variation that warrants attention. Like slowing down at a yellow light, this coding invites us to assess how we can better support or compensate for the variation to maintain balance.

- **Red coding (variant SNPs)** may indicate a greater need for intervention or support, as this variation can significantly impact gene function. A "red light" encourages us to "full stop" and focus on strategies to influence gene expression positively.

Note that very occasionally, variant SNPs (coded red) are the trait providing the most benefit, and normal SNPs (coded green) indicate a need for more significant intervention. For the gene codings covered in this book, please see the SNP Appendix.

Example of SNP Combinations

Here is an example of the various combinations of SNPs you could get from your parents if there is a SNP whose base is A for normal and C for variant:

- If both parents are AA, then you will be AA (normal or "green")

- If both parents are CC, then you will be CC (variant or "red")

- If one parent is AA and the other is CC, then you will be AC (heterozygous or "yellow")

- If one parent is AA and the other is AC, then you will be either AA or AC

- If one parent is AC and another parent is CC, then you will be either CC or AC

- And if both parents are AC, then you will be either AA, AC, or CC

Why Do SNPs Matter?

Most SNPs do not affect health, but some can impact wellness outcomes. While being "normal" might be more common than being "variant," changes that have occurred through evolution in the human race have always happened for a reason.

Think, for example, about grasshoppers. Some grasshoppers are green, and some brown. They usually change color over several generations. The reason for those changes? This allows the grasshopper to better hide from predators. The easiest way to do this is to be the same color as their environment. Does the environment change? Well, yes. There might be more green plants in the rainy season than in the dry season; therefore, it is likely more advantageous to be green in the rainy season. When most grasshoppers are green, that is the "normal" gene, and brown is the "variant." Luckily for grasshoppers, they reproduce quickly and produce thousands of eggs. Those evolutionary changes in insects can happen rapidly. In the dry season, the opposite might be true. A "normal" gene might be brown, and a "variant" gene might be green. Why the change? All organisms on the planet want to survive, and this has to do with environmental conditions.

While human genes cannot evolve as quickly as grasshoppers', we, too, have been amazingly made. As nutritionists specializing in the analyzing and interpreting of genetic data, we align with the broader view that genetic diversity contributes to human adaptability and that neurodivergent traits aren't just deviations but could represent adaptations that were, and continue to be, advantageous in specific environments.

In other words, the differences between typical and neurodivergent brain functioning can be considered creative adaptations—unique ways of responding to diverse environmental challenges and opportunities.

As parents of ADHD children, one of the primary goals is to honor those divergent brain adaptations while also giving our children the greatest chance of success in various essential areas of life by teaching them how to manage situations where those differences (e.g., a green body) might be an environmental mismatch (e.g., the dry season).

ADHD is highly heritable, meaning it often runs in families. When we talk about ADHD and genetics, however, it's important to remember that there isn't a single gene responsible for ADHD, and all studies looking to identify an exact gene or genes that cause ADHD have been inconclusive. Several genome mega-analyses that we have found in the literature, though, have identified specific genetic variations that predispose to ADHD.

SNPs matter because ADHD, influenced by many genes and their specific SNPs, can manifest very differently across individuals. Understanding which SNPs are involved in ADHD allows for a more individualized treatment approach, even without DNA testing.

Genes that Contribute to ADHD

Many genes can contribute to ADHD symptoms, and we'll discuss them throughout the book's seven Core Steps. Currently, the most commonly identified genes in ADHD research include **MTHFR, DRD4**, and **SL6A3** (also known as **DAT1**). MTHFR is involved in methylation, a process affecting neurotransmitter production and function. DRD4 and SL6A3 are linked to the dopamine receptors, which play a crucial role in desire, attention, and reward processing.

While we wish it were as simple as examining three SNPs to determine contributing factors to ADHD symptoms (or most any other condition, for that matter), this is far from reality. When we work with clients, we analyze about 70 genes to understand better the factors contributing to their health challenges.

That is why, while MTHFR often gets attention, looking at it in isolation isn't helpful. Methylation affects many other genes, like sticky notes in your DNA highlighting particular instructions. But focusing solely on MTHFR also overlooks the numerous other genes affecting neurotransmitter pathways, stress response, sleep, and detoxification—ADHD is a complex condition.

Through years of teaching clients how to "reset" their genes (i.e., positively impact gene expression), we've learned you cannot treat methylation issues until you address inflammation and stress. Otherwise, methylation could be overstimulated. So, while genes alone don't provide all the answers, they offer important clues about wellness. Their interactivity can seem overwhelming, but it also provides an array of starting points for supporting your child.

Start with one Step at a time—diet, sleep, movement, or stress management, for example—and build on it based on what feels most manageable for your child.

The World of Epigenetics

Epigenetics, a term coined by Conrad Waddington in the 1940s, refers to changes in gene expression without altering the DNA sequence itself. Think of genes as light bulbs and epigenetic factors as switches, turning them on, off, or dimming their expression. Environmental factors—nutritional intake, exercise, and toxic load—flip or rotate these switches, affecting how genes express themselves. In ADHD, epigenetics helps explain why two people with the same genetic makeup can have different symptoms based on their environments.

Ongoing genetic research holds immense potential for improving ADHD treatments. In our work with clients and group participants, we currently analyze genetic data to provide specialized wellness programs, but future research may allow for even more personalized, effective treatments.

ADHD Gifts

When thinking about ADHD, the focus is often on challenges, but let's also consider the strengths. People with ADHD frequently display remarkable creativity, boundless enthusiasm, and an ability to think outside the box. Their minds can often be on the go—full of ideas, making connections others miss. This unique thinking can lead to innovative solutions and problem-solving, invaluable skills in many areas of life.

While children with ADHD may struggle with attentiveness, their focus can dramatically sharpen when they engage in something they're enthusiastic about. Their high energy, often seen as hyperactivity, can be a significant plus when channeled into activities requiring passion and drive. Impulsivity, frequently viewed as a challenge, can also be a strength—spontaneity can lead to exciting opportunities and experiences.

As children learn to navigate situations that don't align with their ADHD brains, they develop perseverance, adaptability, and problem-solving skills. It is essential to recognize and celebrate these strengths.

Think of people like Albert Einstein, Walt Disney, Bill Gates, Michael Phelps, and Emma Watson. They've all been diagnosed with ADHD. Their success stories remind us that ADHD is about difference, not deficit, and offer an opportunity to change the narrative about it.

Once you identify your child's strengths, nurture them into practical skills. Encourage creativity through drawing, baking, writing, or building projects. These hone your child's inventive skills and give them a productive outlet. High energy can be channeled into physical activities your child enjoys, building self-esteem and creating opportunities for social interaction through teamwork or classes.

As a final point, based on the fact that ADHD presents differently in different people, understand that your child's ADHD symptoms will be unique to them. Some children may experience inattentiveness and hyperactivity, while others struggle with intrusive thoughts, overthinking, or a mix of both. While some children retreat inward, others may be highly physical or aggressive.

Focusing on your child's strengths and addressing their challenges provides a positive framework for helping them thrive.

TRAVELER ASSISTANCE

This chapter's Traveler Assistance will discuss whether you must have your child's DNA tested before using epigenetic "hacks."

In short ... no! At least initially.

However, in the long term, you may decide to proceed with testing, as accessing your child's genetic information will vastly improve your ability to use our recommendations effectively. You will clearly see which genes are variant and better know which Step's suggestions will best support your child's wellness journey. Whenever possible, we suggest getting DNA tested and using a fuller-spectrum test (e.g., Ultimate Genomic kit from https://dnaallure.com/test.html or 23and-Me®'s Health and Ancestry kit) instead of simply a genetic test for medication matches.

Why is that? You can access far more helpful data with a broader test.

GeneSight vs. 23andMe: A Simplified Comparison

GeneSight

GeneSight is a pharmacogenomic test designed to help healthcare providers optimize medication choices for mental health conditions. It analyzes specific genes related to drug metabolism and response, categorizing medications into those to use as directed, those to use with caution, and those likely to cause issues. The test focuses on genes like CYP2D6 (drug metabolism) and COMT (among other tasks, dopamine regulation), among others, and is primarily used for conditions like depression, anxiety, ADHD, and bipolar disorder.

Access: Requires a doctor's order.

Target Group: Mostly adults and adolescents aged 13+.

Cost: GeneSight can be expensive (at the time of publishing, $330US), but many insurance plans in the US partially cover the cost.

Accuracy: Backed by scientific research, it aids decision-making but isn't a diagnostic tool.

Genes Examined: Specific genes involved in the metabolism of medications and the body's response to them. These include genes related to:

- **Cytochrome P450 Enzymes** (e.g., CYP2D6, CYP2C19): Impact the metabolism of many psychiatric medications.

- **Serotonin Transporter Gene** (SLC6A4): Affects serotonin reuptake inhibitors' efficacy and tolerability.

- **Serotonin Receptor Gene** (HTR2A): Plays a role in the response to certain antidepressants.

- **COMT (Catechol-O-methyltransferase)**: Involved in dopamine metabolism, relevant for ADHD and other conditions.

- **ADRA2A (Alpha-2A adrenergic receptor)**: Associated with response to stimulant medications for ADHD.

Sample Collection: A cheek swab.

Interpretation: The provider reviews the results and discusses the implications with the patient.

Availability: Mostly in the US, with limited options in Canada and Europe.

23andMe

23andMe offers consumer-oriented DNA testing focused on ancestry, health traits, and some genetic predispositions. It uses a genotyping process to analyze a curated selection of genetic markers (SNPs), providing insights into health risks, ancestry, and selected traits.

Access: Available directly to consumers in the US, Canada, and some European countries.

Target Group: Anyone interested in their health and ancestry information.

Cost: The Health and Ancestry kit is the version most used by health practitioners. It typically costs about $229 (US) but is often sold for much less.

Accuracy: 23andMe uses a robust genotyping technology to analyze specific single-nucleotide polymorphisms (SNPs). The process is highly accurate for the selected genetic variants it examines.

Genes Examined: Though 23andMe examines far more genes than GeneSight, it still examines only a small fraction of your DNA (~600,000 SNPs) out of ~3 billion base pairs and does not provide information on rare variants.

It does, however, cover the primary genes covered by GeneSight and many, many more, including genes related to:

- **Metabolism Genes**: How you metabolize food intake, ideal feeding window.

- **Macronutrients**: Informs recommended amount of protein, fat, and carbohydrate intake.

- **Neurotransmitter Genes**: Looks at genes related to dopamine, serotonin, and stress responses.

- **Exercise Genes**: Best type of exercise. Exercise recovery.

- **Sleep Genes**: These cover genes related to sleep and circadian rhythm.

- **Detoxification Genes**: Looks at whether your detoxification pathways need support.

- **Inflammation Genes**: Reviews your inflammation responses and, if required, how to support them.

Sample Collection: A spit test.

Interpretation: The material provided by 23andMe is best for general health and ancestry insights, not clinical decision-making. However, the raw DNA data that can be downloaded from 23andMe can, as with dnaallure's data, be used with the GeneRx program by specifically trained MDs, NDs, nutritionists, and other healthcare practitioners to analyze and interpret a range of genes to create a comprehensive wellness plan.

Accessibility: Available directly to consumers in the US, Canada, and some European countries.

If your priority is medication guidance for ADHD or other mental health conditions for adults or children over the age of about 13, GeneSight provides clinical utility. For general genetic exploration or ancestry, 23andMe offers a more accessible and cost-effective option and provides the raw DNA data for much more in-depth analysis and interpretation. If data privacy and security are of concern, note that at the time of this book's publication, you can:

Opt-Out of Research: You can choose whether or not your genetic and survey data are included in research studies conducted by 23andMe or third-party partners.

Control Data Sharing: Users can decide whether to share their data with specific services, such as pharmaceutical partners, or keep it strictly within 23andMe.

Request Anonymity: Research data is de-identified, meaning it is stripped of personally identifiable information before being shared or analyzed.

You can also choose to delete your account at any time, which includes the deletion of genetic information from 23andMe systems.

A final note on DNAAllure and the various DNA testing options: Some time ago, our clients were having difficulty downloading their raw data from 23andMe or accessing 23andMe in certain locations. Dr. Kendall-Reed had a private lab in Canada create a DNA kit (that can be sent worldwide via FedEx) to test the genes used in the GeneRx platform specifically. The genes analyzed in this lab's Ultimate Genomics kit are used in the GeneRX platform to obtain a comprehensive 60+-page report addressing the genes that can give us insight into ADHD and other health challenges. In our practices, we use primarily DNAAllure and 23andMe raw data.

For many parents, deciding to test their child's DNA can be difficult. Getting fully informed consent from a child or teen is impossible since they can't grasp the whole concept of DNA or the testing implications. For parents who decide to skip testing, the recommendations in this book will involve assessing their child's symptoms to match the SNPs described and adjusting lifestyle factors accordingly.

Another path starts with our general recommendations and makes adjustments through trial and error—tweaking protein intake, adjusting bedtimes, trying different exercise styles, and introducing supplements one at a time—to see what works best for their child.

However, with the information from DNA testing, an individual child's specific SNPs are clearly identified, and parents can go directly to implementing the most impactful solutions. Note: Only health practitioners trained in specific software can utilize the data in DNAAllure's results, and they will not be quite as comprehensive as through 23andMe. In addition, if you decide to do the DNA Allure test, you will need practitioner information: please contact us (info@inbalancelm.com) for our Clinic details.

I (Brenda) didn't have Rachel's DNA tested when she was a child dealing with ADHD; the technology didn't exist at the time. But as a social worker, nutritionist, and bit of a hippie earth-mama, our family's approach to eating, moving, sleeping, and self-regulating supported her well, even without a diagnosis or knowing her specific SNPs. The refined version of this approach is laid out in our general suggestions. As a young adult, Rachel has chosen to have her DNA tested, which has allowed us to fine-tune strategies. Still, much of what we've learned has only confirmed what we were already doing.

Any of these approaches will help you begin to personalize your child's wellness. They will support your child's ADHD strengths while improving their responses in situations that don't match well with how their brain functions.

DNA Testing vs. Blood Tests

A final note on the difference between a DNA test and a blood test: We got our DNA from our parents the minute our dad's sperm fertilized our mom's egg. This DNA has never changed and will never change until our last day on the planet. The difference between a DNA test and a blood test is that most blood tests evaluate what is happening when the blood is drawn.

Blood tests certainly have a role in wellness evaluation, but note that, depending upon what you are testing, you could require endless blood tests throughout your life. In contrast, you will only ever need one DNA test.

If DNA Doesn't Change, What's a "Reset?"

To make the science of epigenetics more relatable (and to emphasize the powerful idea that changes in lifestyle, environment, and behavior can positively influence genetic expression!), we sometimes mention a gene reset or resetting a gene.

It reminds you and your child that you have some control over your biology and encourages you to take actionable steps to manage and improve your physical and emotional wellness.

Be aware, however, that as catchy and easy to remember as "gene reset" is, we don't want to oversimplify gene expression or suggest a level of permanence (i.e., eat this way, exercise like this, or detox this way for a month, and all your child's more challenging ADHD behaviors will be resolved).

Epigenetic change is generally an ongoing, cumulative process influenced by multiple factors (thus, the seven Steps in this book). You can't rewrite your DNA. You can, however, put patterns into place that improve gene expression while not necessarily erasing all past effects.

So, while we'll occasionally use the term gene reset, note that we're referring to the complex and dynamic nuanced process of epigenetic regulation—gene optimization.

REST STOP

REST STOP

		WHAT: Ask questions and be present with answers. WHY: Gain tools to allow deeper responses.
	WHAT & WHY	
	REST - 10 MIN. OF CALM	10 minutes of *calm* to REST with the questions. Review your notes, ponder the questions.
	STOP - 10 MIN. OF QUIET	10 minutes of *quiet* to STOP for the answers. Keep your mind clear and open. Jot down responses.

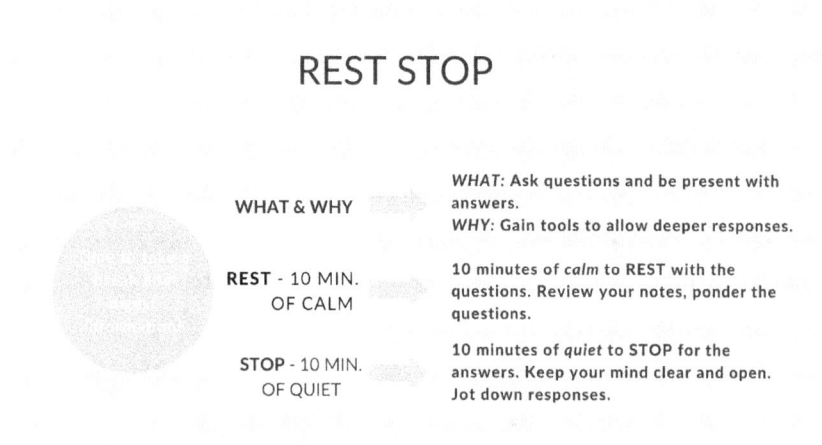

It's time for parents to take a break and digest information! Per the diagram, take 10 minutes of calm to Rest with the following questions:

1. **Gifts and Challenges:** Have I been able to inventory my child's ADHD gifts and challenges realistically?

2. **Where Do I Land?:** Do I tend to focus on one or the other category? If so, why?

Next, Stop for 10 minutes of quiet (sitting or slowly walking). Keep your mind as clear and open as possible, and just listen. Jot down thoughts in your parents' Trip Log or tell Siri to "make a note" of any responses that may arise. Because you've taken time to ponder calmly and quietly, these responses will most likely be less off-the-cuff and from a deeper level. They can give you clues as to the reasons behind your answers! Those clues, in turn, will reveal potential problematic thinking and can provide great direction on moving forward with the recommendations in this Step that would be the easiest to implement or fit best for your family!

ROADWORK

Discover Your Strengths

Materials:

- A large sheet of paper

- Colored markers, crayons, and optional stickers

Directions:

1. **Have Your Child Draw a Big Circle** in the center of the paper. Have them write their name in the middle.

2. **Around the Circle,** have them draw smaller circles and help them label them with different strengths (e.g., creativity, problem-solving, enthusiasm).

3. **Inside Each Small Circle,** write down activities that can help develop these strengths (e.g., drawing, building projects, role-playing games).

4. **Decorate the Chart** with stickers or colors to make it visually appealing and fun for your child. Hang it in a common area where everyone can see and add to it over time.

This activity helps you and your child visualize strengths and brainstorm ways to cultivate them. It turns abstract concepts into concrete actions and reminds you of your child's unique abilities and potential.

SOUVENIR

After wading through the science-heavy parts of this chapter, it's time to celebrate! Grab a sparkling water and toast to your progress.

We'd also like to give you a helpful checklist for preparing for consultations to ease the stress of meeting new healthcare providers.

Preparing for Consultations: A Checklist

- **Medical Records**: Bring your child's medical history, including past diagnoses, treatments, and medications.

- **Symptom List**: Document all symptoms, even those that seem unrelated to ADHD.

- **Questions**: Prepare questions like, "How can diet affect my child's behavior?" or "What are the side effects of this medication?"

- **Medication List**: Include medications and supplements.

- **Behavioral Observations**: Note any patterns, such as times when symptoms worsen.

- **Communication Plan**: Ensure all providers agree to collaborate on a cohesive treatment plan.

Chapter 3

ADHD Primer - Early Years to Longer Term and Diagnosis

"I was a hyperactive child. I am still a hyperactive adult. I know that. My kid is the same as me."

- Diego, a client of Alicia's

INFORMATION CENTER

Imagine you're at a playground, watching your 3-year-old dart from the sandbox to the slide, their energy seemingly endless. While other parents chat about their latest Netflix viewing, your mind is focused on familiar behaviors: constant movement, grabbing toys from other children, inability to sit still, and constant interruptions. These actions might be more than toddler antics—they could be early signs of ADHD.

ADHD Across the Lifespan: From Toddlers to Adults

Recognizing ADHD in toddlers can be challenging. The Mayo Clinic notes that it's hard to diagnose in toddlers or preschoolers because other factors, like hearing loss or speech delays, may mimic ADHD symptoms. Inattention and impulsivity are often typical for toddlers, so early symptoms such as excessive fidgeting, obsessiveness, or uncontrollableness can be mistaken for typical behavior.

As children grow, ADHD traits like inattention, hyperactivity, and impulsivity become clearer. The challenge is distinguishing an active, spirited child from one with ADHD. Conversely, girls or boys with a quieter nature often go undiagnosed. Their symptoms can manifest as daydreaming or inattentiveness rather than the more noticeable hyperactivity frequently seen in boys or more active girls.

For teens, ADHD's challenges shift. Adolescence brings academic pressures and social dynamics that can magnify ADHD symptoms. Organizational struggles, poor time management, and difficulty focusing can lead to underachievement. Co-occurring conditions like depression or anxiety may complicate the situation. Intrusive thoughts and overthinking, quieter aspects of ADHD, also become more apparent, affecting self-esteem, emotional regulation, and social interactions.

Family communication can become strained during these years. Adolescence inherently brings challenges, but ADHD can intensify them.

Having a Teenager With ADHD in Real Life

I (Brenda) recall heated conversations with my daughter Rachel when she was a teenager, who, unbeknownst to us at the time, had ADHD. She was often impatient with my communication, and I was frustrated by her shortness and seeming indifference. Our discussions frequently escalated, ending in outbursts. Eventually, during a calmer moment, we devised a "secret handshake" to signal when we needed a brief timeout to clear our heads. This simple gesture of linking our pinkie fingers helped us know it was time for a break. We used it to avoid further escalation, for a time-out, and to come back together to, in most instances, communicate more effectively.

Effective Parenting, which I (Alicia) am trained in, offers similar tools for fostering communication and trust. In this chapter's Traveler Assistance, I'll show you how to create a Family Code that can help with communication before, during, and after the teenage years.

Beyond Adolescence

ADHD often persists into adulthood, though its symptoms may evolve. Hyperactivity may diminish, but focus, impulsivity, and executive function challenges remain. Adults with ADHD frequently struggle with tasks requiring sustained attention, like managing finances or meeting deadlines. Restlessness, boredom, and a tendency to interrupt conversations can affect personal and professional relationships.

The transition to adulthood brings new responsibilities, and coping mechanisms that were effective in school may not translate to work or an independent home life. About 50% of children diagnosed with ADHD continue to experience symptoms as adults, making lifelong recognition and treatment crucial for achieving potential and well-being.

Dr. Greenblatt emphasized in a recent webinar that untreated ADHD can negatively impact career, self-esteem, relationships, academic achievement, and stress levels.

A father from our community confirmed the real-life results of Dr. Greenblatt's statement when he continued his quote from the beginning of this chapter: "I was a hyperactive child, I know that. My kid is the same as me. And as an adult, I struggle with keeping my job and staying focused. I get bored very easily, and I'd rather play soccer with my child than be a breadwinner." Diego's comments highlight the importance of monitoring and adapting treatment strategies from childhood through adulthood.

It's Time for Undergraduate Studies, Now What?

AKA to apply for or not apply for academic accommodations.

Maya, a vibrant teen with ADHD, struggled with attention in her early years. As she entered adolescence, intrusive thoughts and anxiety worsened. Her parents worked with healthcare providers to adjust her treatment, incorporating cognitive-behavioral therapy and modifying her school environment to reduce distractions. Now preparing for college, Maya has worked with the school's Center for Accessible Learning to secure extended exam time and a notetaker, giving her the best chance for success.

If you or your child are still deciding whether to pursue academic accommodations, please accept our encouragement to explore the possibility. Brenda and Alicia have both encountered accommodations in higher education: Brenda worked in a university department that determined and administered them, and Alicia often encounters students with accommodations in the university courses she teaches.

These "leveling of the playing field" accommodations are becoming much more common and well-accepted practices, and they can be very beneficial for your child academically, mentally, and emotionally.

One summer, my (Brenda) husband, Mark, and I spent a week canoeing the Turner Lake Chain in BC's interior. Determining the proper trails to follow, paddling through rapids, and portaging over rough terrain was exhilarating, challenging, and wearying. In many ways, navigating ADHD through the different stages of life is very similar to that trip.

The key is to stay vigilant, be adaptive, and seek the resources and support to make the journey smoother. On a short side note? Paddling with friends who've previously taken the journey can also be helpful!

The Role of Environment in ADHD Expression

When it comes to ADHD, the debate between nature and nurture can feel like a tug-of-war. On one side, experts like Dr. Gabor Maté, in *Scattered Minds*, emphasize nurture. Dr. Maté argues that while there may be a genetic susceptibility to ADHD, it is rooted in multigenerational family stress and disturbed social conditions. ADHD, in his view, doesn't have to be a fixed, lifelong condition but is influenced by life experiences and family dynamics. This perspective underscores improving the child's environment, reducing stress, and promoting emotional healing over labeling or diagnosis.

Similarly, Dr. Gordon Neufeld doesn't view ADHD as primarily neurological. He suggests that many attention issues, including ADHD, stem from emotional development, attachment, and maturation problems.

Conversely, practitioners like Dr. Russell Barkley emphasize genetic predispositions rather than environmental factors like parenting style. He sees ADHD as a neurodevelopmental disorder with a strong genetic component and advocates structured interventions and evidence-based treatments to manage symptoms.

These perspectives all have valid points and supportive research: genetics provides the blueprint for how a brain, hormones, and responses to things like diet, activity, or supplements work; environment plays a decisive role in either exacerbating or mitigating symptoms.

Where We Land in the ADHD Tug-of-War

Where are we in the nature vs. nurture tug-of-war? We're somewhere in the middle, recognizing that ADHD is both a genetic and environmental condition. We tend to align more with Dr. Neufeld's view, with our adaptation being to layer genetics as a foundation. We believe many ADHD symptoms are not permanent. Addressing emotional and developmental causes can help children develop more vigorous attention over time.

However, we also emphasize genetics more than Dr. Maté or Dr. Neufeld, seeing genetic challenges as co-contributors to ADHD symptoms. A holistic approach is needed, as solely focusing on emotional or genetic factors won't fully address ADHD behaviors. We feel that understanding how genes influence ADHD symptoms, alongside the role of environment, offers a more balanced approach to managing ADHD.

By tackling both contributing sets of factors, you allow your child to grow and evolve into their best possible genuine self. You don't strip them of true aspects of their neurodiversity; you provide them with the tools to be a better match for challenging situations in which they must be present successfully.

The environmental triggers we discuss in this book can significantly influence how ADHD symptoms manifest. For example, diet can either calm or worsen behavior. A diet high in ultra-processed foods with sugar and additives can increase hyperactivity, while one rich in omega-3s and whole foods may improve brain function.

Stress is another critical factor. High-stress environments, at home or school, can exacerbate symptoms. Exposure to toxins like lead or chemicals and lack of physical activity also impact ADHD symptoms. These environmental factors interact with genetic predispositions, creating a complex web of influences that make each child's ADHD experience unique.

Attachment and Authenticity

Creating a nurturing environment can ease many ADHD challenges. Dr. Maté's work emphasizes the importance of attachment and authenticity at home and school. A securely attached child who feels understood is more likely to thrive. This means fostering a home environment where your child can express emotions freely and a school that meets their unique needs. Positive reinforcement, structured routines, and open communication are essential to creating stability, reducing anxiety, and improving behavior.

When we come to one of our Supplemental Essentials—ADHD Family Dynamics—and look at Completing the Stress Cycle, we can see that many of the recommendations are best implemented with a strong and healthy parental connection.

A Personalized ADHD Approach

Lifestyle choices are crucial to managing ADHD. A personalized diet, regular sleep patterns, and consistent exercise are foundational.

- Diet affects neurotransmitter function, influencing attention and behavior.

- Sleep is critical for brain health, and irregular patterns can worsen symptoms.

- Exercise helps regulate dopamine and norepinephrine, improving focus and reducing impulsivity.

- Detoxifying your home by reducing harmful chemicals can make a noticeable impact on overall wellness.

These lifestyle choices minimize situational mismatches while honoring your child's uniqueness, allowing their best self to emerge.

Diagnosing ADHD: Signs, Symptoms, and Assessments

Diagnosing ADHD involves more than noticing that your child has trouble sitting still or paying attention. The DSM-5 (Diagnostic and Statistical Manual of Mental Disorders, Fifth Edition) outlines the criteria, details of which can be found in our Diagnosing ADHD Appendix. For example, from the diagnostic criteria for ADHD, where adults need five inattention and/or hyperactivity-impulsivity symptoms, though undiagnosed, I (Alicia) have ten.

When ADHD Might Not Be ADHD

Note, too, that other conditions and situations can foster ADHD-like symptoms. These include learning disorders, intellectual disabilities, Sensory Processing Disorder, Autism Spectrum Disorder, and mental and emotional health issues such as anxiety, depression, bipolar disorder, or Oppositional Defiant Disorder.

Health challenges such as sleep disorders, thyroid dysfunction, epilepsy, PANDAS/PANS (Pediatric Autoimmune Neuropsychiatric Disorders Associated with Streptococcal Infections), Auditory Processing Disorder, heavy metals exposure, and vision or hearing problems can cause ADHD-like symptoms.

Your child may be experiencing dietary issues such as allergies or nutrient deficiencies or have side effects due to certain medications and, again, be presenting with ADHD symptoms.

It's also important to consider stress and trauma issues, either physical or emotional, that can lead to symptoms that resemble ADHD symptoms. These factors can have a significant impact and should not be overlooked.

Given the wide range of conditions that can present with ADHD symptoms, it's important to have a thorough and multifaceted assessment by several different healthcare professionals. This approach ensures that other possibilities are ruled out, providing a sense of security and an accurate diagnosis.

Finally, given this book's focus on genetics, it makes sense to get a blueprint of your child's DNA and a complete set of assessments. This can give a great deal of insight into where ADHD symptoms may be arising in the body's many systems.

Early Diagnosis

An early, accurate diagnosis of ADHD—between the ages of 4 and 7—can significantly benefit both a child and their family. I (Brenda) certainly wish we'd had Rachel's diagnosis at a much earlier age, and I'm very glad that before Rachel was diagnosed, many of the epigenetic suggestions we make in this book were regular parts of our household practices for all our children!

Understanding what your child is dealing with allows you to implement effective strategies, reducing frustration and helplessness. Early diagnosis opens doors to interventions—behavioral therapies, educational accommodations, dietary changes, sleep support, supplements, and medication, if appropriate—that can improve outcomes. It's not just about managing symptoms but fostering your child's ability to navigate the world in a way that works for them.

Imagine you suspect your child has ADHD and consult a healthcare provider for an assessment, including rating scales, behavioral tests, and teacher input. The diagnosis is confirmed, and things start making sense. The challenges are rooted in a neurodevelopmental difference, and while shifts in parenting approach can significantly help your child, you did not cause their ADHD by the way you parent. With this understanding, you can implement tailored strategies like structured routines, specialized educational support, and possibly treatment. The diagnosis becomes a tool for better management, not a limiting label.

Between the ages of 3 and 12, the brain is especially receptive to forming new connections and reorganizing synapses—a process known as neuroplasticity. During this period of heightened neuroplasticity, the brain can adapt and develop new pathways in response to interventions, making it an ideal time for personalized, integrated support. However, for this potential to be fully realized, the accuracy of the diagnosis is crucial. Misdiagnosing or unnecessarily medicating a child could lead to unintended side effects, potentially hindering rather than supporting their development. Likewise, if medication could prove beneficial and isn't prescribed, behavioral and emotional progress can be hampered. (More on this under Medical and Alternative Treatments for ADHD.)

Early diagnosis also helps in setting realistic goals and expectations. A clearer understanding of your child's strengths and challenges allows you to work with educators and healthcare providers to develop individualized education plans (IEPs) or other accommodations. This proactive approach can prevent potential negative consequences of untreated ADHD, such as academic underachievement, low self-esteem, and social difficulties. It also allows for ongoing monitoring and adjustments to the treatment plan as your child grows. Early and accurate diagnosis can lead to better outcomes in the long run.

Being diagnosed with ADHD can also have its own set of benefits. Knowing what your child is dealing with allows you to tailor strategies that work specifically for them. It opens doors to resources and accommodations that can significantly impact their academic and social lives. Understanding ADHD can also help you appreciate your child's unique strengths, like creativity and varied approaches to a topic or situation. These qualities can be nurtured and celebrated.

While in the past (and even sometimes today), getting a diagnosis of ADHD could feel like a limiting factor in potential or a "label" that could potentially foster exclusion or bullying, we like to think of diagnosis as a first step in understanding and in positive movement forward.

TRAVELER ASSISTANCE

A family code or set of values can help create a framework for household rules, family time, play, chores, and general interactions. Here's a **Creating a Family Code** activity I (Alicia) learned as an Effective Parenting Coach:

Creating a Family Code (from Effective Parenting, Niños de Ahora, Mexico)
Four things to remember before creating your Family Code:

1. The goal is to support each other, not hurt anyone's feelings.

2. Treat everyone as equals; for this exercise, being a parent doesn't make you different.

3. Difficult moments help you grow and learn together.

4. Reasoning and many other cognitive abilities develop significantly with age, influencing the capacity to think logically, make decisions, and evaluate consequences. This development can impact emotional regulation, reasonableness, and behavior, particularly during family meetings and planning sessions. For good clues as to what to expect, check the CDC's Developmental Milestones (https://www.cdc.gov/ncbddd/actearly/milestones/index.html).

Let everyone contribute, and be a good listener.

- **Step 1:** List the goals you want to achieve as a family (e.g., "We encourage each other," "We feel safe at home").

- **Step 2:** List daily activities to achieve these goals (e.g., "I'll be present to encourage," "Lots of hugs and kisses").

- **Step 3:** List the values you want to live by (e.g., "I stay calm before responding," "I prioritize family time").

- **Step 4:** Create your family code together. For younger kids, let them draw or express their ideas. Clarify instead of rejecting suggestions.

Make your code visible (e.g., post it on the fridge or create a framed picture). Use it as a guide when things don't go according to code. If it's not working, redo it with your family.

Example Family Code:

- We respect each other without arguing, shouting, or insulting.

- We are good listeners.

- We give hugs often to stay present with others.

- Mom and Dad calmly listen and don't have loud arguments.

- We work to be happy and support each other.

- We take care of our daily healthy habits (e.g., eating, sleeping, moving).

REST STOP

It's time for parents to take a break and digest information! Take 10 minutes of calm to Rest with the following questions:

1. **Nature vs. Nurture:** Where have I been on the sliding scale of what causes ADHD, with one end primarily genetic and the other primarily environmental?

2. **Thinking Shifts:** Have I moved on that scale at all? If so, in which

direction and why? If not, why not?

Next, Stop for 10 minutes of quiet (sitting or slowly walking). Keep your mind as clear and open as possible, and just listen. Jot down or tell Siri to "make a note" of any responses that may arise. Because you've taken time to ponder calmly and quietly, these responses will most likely be less off-the-cuff and from a deeper level. They can give you clues as to the reasons behind your answers! Those clues, in turn, will reveal potential problematic thinking and can provide great direction on moving forward with the recommendations in this Step that would be the easiest to implement or fit best for your family!

ROADWORK

For your Roadwork in this chapter, we suggest you track your child's various behaviors and symptoms, noting whether you can discern triggers and practices that support your child's ability to express their diversity and strengths while giving them tools to handle situational mismatches.

We'll also touch on ADHD Burnout as a condition to watch for in the journaling.

Daily Symptom Tracker
Materials:

- A notebook or digital device

- Pen

Directions:

1. **Create Sections:** Divide your page into sections for different times of the day (morning, afternoon, evening).

2. **Note Symptoms:** Jot down any ADHD symptoms you observe in your child during these times. Be specific—note the symptoms and activity your child was doing.

3. **Identify Triggers:** Look for patterns or triggers. Does your child get more fidgety before lunch or after eating certain foods? Is focusing a challenge after screen time?

4. **Reflect:** At the end of the week, review your notes. Discuss any patterns with your child and your child's healthcare provider to adjust strategies or treatments as needed.

This simple activity helps you track your child's symptoms, spot patterns, and identify what works best.

ADHD Burnout

Note that various elements can contribute to a change in your child's behavior, many of which we'll discuss in this book. Be aware, however, that a concept called ADHD burnout may be a factor. While not a medical diagnosis, ADHD burnout refers to the physical, emotional, and mental exhaustion that can be experienced by those diagnosed with ADHD as they attempt to manage the challenges of scenarios where their brain functioning is mismatched with their situation.

Contributing factors to ADHD burnout can be:

- **Perfectionism:** Many times, children with ADHD are wired to strive for perfection and have great difficulty accepting less than that in their efforts. This trait can create significant pressure.

- **Overcommitment:** Children with ADHD can take on an excessive amount of tasks, leading to an equally excessive amount of overload.

- **ADHD Masking:** Hiding or downplaying ADHD behaviors in an attempt to "fit in" to an environment can lead to anxiety and fatigue.

When journaling your child's triggers and response behaviors, consider whether perfectionism, overcommitment, or masking may be at play. If so, addressing some of these root characteristics can help you and your child minimize unhelpful responses (e.g., constant dopamine-seeking patterns).

SOUVENIR

For this Step's Souvenir, we'll reference the previous Traveler Assistance and cover some ways my (Brenda's) family has marked our family code.

- We've shared family genealogies and values passed down through generations.

- I commissioned a pictorial family tree for my husband on our anniversary.

- During a family vacation, we visited Ellis Island and had a family name history created for my mother's maiden name, Sloan.

But perhaps the most meaningful is our family values wall, created with Sid Dickens' Memory Blocks. We chose tiles representing our values, and later, one of our adult children and his wife added a tile. Those tiles hang in our living room, reminding us of our values and motivating us to live by them.

Alicia and I encourage you to create your own Family Code and display it as a daily inspiration for your family.

Now, let's move on to how you can optimize your child's nutrition to support their ADHD management.

Chapter 4

Core Step One - Eat

"In terms of "personal health," nutrigenomics can recommend a diet that minimizes risks imparted by an individual's genotype."
- Dr. Penny Kendall-Reed

SUMMARY - Travel Size Version

It's 7 AM, and you're trying to get breakfast ready while your child, who has already moved through three different play areas, leaving a mountain of material for "clean-up" time, asks for pancakes and syrup. You know that what they eat can make a difference, but trying to navigate the vast amounts of nutritional advice found online or on your local big-box bookstore shelves feels like hacking through a jungle ... with a plastic spoon! This chapter is your clear pathway forward.

Tips on Understanding Our Gene References

Before we explore the genes that affect your child's metabolism and their response to macronutrients (proteins, fats, and carbohydrates), we'll provide some insight into how we refer to genes.

Nutrition's Role in Managing ADHD

We'll help you understand how food can either fuel your child's stormy challenges or calm them.

We'll cover genes that determine your child's optimal food plan and best feeding window. Then, we'll explain how to interpret that info with or even without DNA testing.

Because many parents report their children are picky eaters, we'll start by exploring why picky eating happens and what to do about it.

The Massive Importance of Micronutrients

Next, we'll explore the crucial role of vitamins and minerals in managing ADHD symptoms. If macronutrients are the brain's fuel, micronutrients like omega-3 fatty acids, magnesium, and zinc are the maintenance crew, ensuring everything runs smoothly.

In BALANCE Food Pyramid

This pyramid, which I (Brenda) created more than a decade ago, serves as a blueprint for balanced nutrition. At its foundation, you'll find BALANCE: Body Type, Attitude, Laughter and play, Activity, a good Night's sleep, Clean water, and Eating for Health.

Food Plans

Various dietary plans help manage ADHD symptoms. We'll discuss feeding windows, meal timing, and elimination diets, which can help reduce hyperactivity and improve focus.

Elimination diets involve removing potential allergens to see if symptoms improve. This detective work helps find what works best for your child, especially if detoxification genes are involved (more on those in Step 4).

Meal Planning

Knowing what nutrients your child needs is one thing; making cohesive, tasty meals is often something altogether different! We'll offer meal planning tips to ensure everyone gets the proper nutrient balance, avoid mealtime meltdowns, and create enjoyable family meals.

Sometimes Foods

No nutrition discussion is complete without "Sometimes Foods," which may not be the healthiest but add joy and celebration. We'll help you understand how genetics, inflammation, and metabolism affect how often Sometimes Foods can be enjoyed with less negative impact.

Supplements

Supplements can fill nutritional gaps. We'll explain how to choose high-quality supplements that complement, rather than replace, a well-rounded diet.

INFORMATION CENTER

Meet Kiran, a seven-year-old with ADHD. His dad noticed Kiran was more focused and less hyperactive when he ate a breakfast of eggs, whole-grain toast, and a piece of fruit. He also saw improvements when they introduced a daily fish oil supplement. Kiran enjoyed a couple of homemade cookies on weekends, but his parents limited sugar intake to once a week, balancing it with options that more suited his dietary needs the rest of the time. Observing Kiran's responses to different foods and adjusting his diet, his parents found a nutritional plan supporting his genetics.

Tips on Understanding Our Gene References and Emphasis

In this chapter, you will encounter several of the first genes we highlight as potentially playing a role in ADHD. These particular genes may help explain whether less-than-optimal nutrition contributes to your child's ADHD symptoms. While we've organized the potential gene factors by Core Step, it's important to remember that these genes don't work in isolation—they interact in complex ways.

Additionally, it's crucial to remember the profound impact of stress and inflammation on gene expression. Regardless of the Core Step being discussed, and even if your child has normal coding for the genes in question, stress and inflammation can significantly alter gene expression, effectively causing up to 90% of genes to behave as if they are variant. This underscores the importance of managing stress and inflammation to support your child's overall well-being.

Lastly, note that we will not include gene or SNP rs numbers—a cataloging method—in the body of the text. If you have DNA testing results for your child and wish to explore specific gene information (including coding) to tailor the book's recommendations, please refer to the SNPs Appendix.

If your child hasn't had DNA testing, review the gene information and note your child's symptoms, then apply the suggestions that seem most relevant and manageable to implement. After 7-10 days of trying a set of recommendations (e.g., for Eat or Sleep Steps), evaluate your child's response. Adjust if needed, and if things are improving, move on to the next set of appropriate suggestions (e.g., Calm or Move Steps). Again, allow for 7-10 days before reevaluating.

Picky and Disordered Eating

Picky eating is typically marked by a child's consistent (or inconsistent) refusal of certain foods or food groups, a strong preference for a limited variety (hello, ketchup!), and reluctance to try new foods. Over time, this restricted diet can lead to nutrient deficiencies and impact growth and physiology.

Sensory sensitivities, temperament, genetics, and environmental factors can influence this behavior. According to one systematic review, picky eating is often found in children whose parents describe them as being "stubborn," "moody," "nervous," and "easily distracted."

Hmmm.

Have you heard those characteristics mentioned before and sometimes linked to children with ADHD? Is it possible there may be some crossover between the many genes that contribute to ADHD behaviors and biological factors that may contribute to picky eating or even, eventually, disordered eating?

Experts certainly think so.

ADHD is increasingly recognized as a risk factor for disordered eating behaviors linked to unique neurobiological and behavioral traits. Impulse control challenges in ADHD can make it harder to resist immediate gratification, such as eating whatever food is available, even when not hungry ("see food, eat food").

Additionally, the brain's reward system, particularly the biochemistry of dopamine, plays a significant role. Dopamine dysregulation in ADHD may lead individuals to seek out highly palatable, sugary, or fatty foods that provide quick dopamine hits, potentially fostering food-hiding behaviors and addictive patterns of eating.

Research has also shown that ADHD traits, such as emotional dysregulation and difficulties with planning, can contribute to binge eating, emotional eating, and even restrictive eating patterns. Dr. Roberto Olivardia, a clinical psychologist and expert on ADHD, emphasizes the connection between ADHD and eating disorders, noting that individuals with ADHD are at increased risk for behaviors like binge eating and night eating syndrome due to these neurobiological vulnerabilities. Addressing these tendencies often takes a multifaceted approach, including behavioral strategies, nutritional education, and emotional regulation techniques.

We agree with these experts, which is why we cover each of those approaches throughout our Steps. Because environment impacts gene expression, with the right Eating, Sleeping, and Calm tools, picky eating can diminish over time, and disordered eating can be minimized. To begin with, however, here are a couple of suggestions to encourage a broader range of food selection.

First, we like Ellyn Satter's Division of Responsibility in Feeding (sDOR). The sDOR is a well-regarded approach that establishes clear roles for parents and children during mealtimes to foster a positive and balanced feeding relationship. According to this model, parents are responsible for deciding *what*, *when*, and *where* food is offered, ensuring that nutritious options are available and con-sistent. Children, in turn, are responsible for choosing *whether* to eat and *how much* to eat from the options provided. This division allows children to develop a healthy relationship with food, promotes self-regulation, and reduces mealtime struggles by respecting children's natural hunger and satiety cues. Satter's website has valuable tips on walking out her approach in real life.

Secondly, we place a high value on modeling the behaviors we'd like children to adopt. This value is not simply because modeling has been a parenting buzzword since the 1960s and goes far beyond the cute instinctual process of a gosling imprinting on the first moving object they see.

Distinct from imprinting (a biologically pre-programmed and time-limited process), modeling is a dynamic and ongoing learning process that allows for tremendous growth, flexibility, and adaptability throughout a person's life.

And while we can look at "buzzwords" with disdain and suspicion, they are sometimes discussed because they result from groundbreaking work, are simple, and are effective!

Modeling has sound backing as an effective parenting strategy for at least three reasons:

1. **Social Learning Theory**: Albert Bandura's Social Learning Theory explains that children learn behaviors by observing and imitating others. Parents and caregivers are primary role models, and their actions serve as a blueprint for children's behavior.

2. **Neurological Basis**: Mirror neurons in the brain enable children to mimic observed behaviors. This biological mechanism makes modeling one of the most natural and effective ways for children to learn.

3. **Consistency and Trust**: Modeling establishes consistency between parents' words and deeds. This alignment fosters trust and credibility, increasing children's likelihood of adopting desired behaviors.

However, back to picky eating! I (Alicia) often hear moms say their kids won't eat vegetables or only want high-starch foods. As you might expect, one suggestion for encouraging kids to eat vegetables or protein is modeling that behavior yourself. One family I worked with saw their daughter go from refusing to eat vegetables to eating broccoli because she saw her mom do it.

Later, in the ADHD Family Dynamics chapter, we discuss behavioral mirroring in terms of parents modeling the completion of the stress cycle. However, the modeling concept applies to virtually all the Steps we cover. Your child is often a reflection of you, especially when they are young. There is a high chance that whatever you do, they will imitate. Along with implementing our other picky eater suggestions, you could ask yourself some questions such as:

- Am I modeling avoidance of certain vegetables, proteins, or healthy fats?

- Am I modeling eating a variety of colors, flavors, and textures?

- Am I modeling ultra-processed food intake?

I (Alicia) once heard picky eater expert Becky Miksic explain that learning to eat and swallow is more complicated than learning to swim because all five senses are involved. If broccoli smells like sulfur or looks overcooked and brown, it's no wonder kids avoid it. Try steaming it briefly to make it a bright green, wait for the smell to fade, add tasty dressing, and tell a fun "broccoli" story to engage them.

In our (Brenda's) household, we addressed pickiness in three ways:

- Our kids helped cook, bake, or prep for dinner. When they chopped mushrooms or set the table, our five were more willing to try what we made.

- We let them express opinions about meals—politely, with thumbs up or down, or a 5-star rating.

- We implemented a household "one taste" rule. Our rationale was that if our kids never again tried zucchini, they might go decades without eating it when they'd actually grown to like it. If it was still a no-go after the taste, they could leave that food on the side of their plate. For each meal, two types of foods (think onions and peppers) could be left on the plate—no harm, no foul.

That meant Mark and I spent many years eating a lot of onions, peppers, zucchini, and mushrooms, but it gave our kids some agency over what they wanted to eat while encouraging them to try new flavors.

For several reasons we'll soon cover both Alicia's and Brenda's households focused on natural, whole-food intake. We are also glad we did because several studies link dietary patterns like "junk food," "processed," "snack," "sweet," and "Western" diets to a higher risk of ADHD.

Nutrition's Role in Managing ADHD Symptoms

Before we discuss the science of nutrition and ADHD, let's review some basics from our decades of experience in nutritional consultation. If you've followed our work, you're already familiar with our 3 Food Foundations and 5 Simple Food Keys.

Apologies in advance if you were hoping we'd changed our stance on good-for-your-body-and-brain food intake and now advocate a lot of ul-tra-processed food and caffeine. It's not going to happen!

THREE FOOD FOUNDATIONS

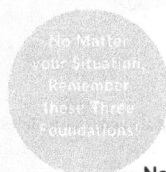

No Matter your Situation, Remember these Three Foundations!

Eat Real Food → Eat things that were meant to be eaten. Preferably fresh and local.

Close to Origin → Eat closer to "back to basics" origins rather than processed or with additives.

No Food Fanaticism → Get help with food addictions and disordered eating.

FIVE FOOD KEYS

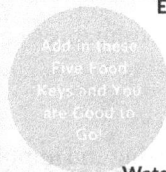

Add in these Five Food Keys and You are Good to Go!

Minimize Refined Foods → Consider white flour and sugar products as rare "Sometimes Foods."

Eat Enough Protein → Each time you eat, include animal or vegetable-sourced protein.

Get Enough Fat → Eat healthy fats and fat-rich foods that have a long history of traditional use.

Watch the Dairy Intake → If tolerated, eat small amounts of cleanly-sourced dairy products.

Increase the Veggies → Eat 6-10 servings of raw and cooked vegetables/day (and a bit of fruit).

If it's been a while since you've thought about protein, fat, and carbohydrates, don't worry—we'll cover them when discussing macronutrient genes.

Metabolic Genes

The **MC4R** gene plays a central role in satiety and controlling food intake. It influences hunger, desire to snack, and body weight. While we're not focused on weight loss here, understanding how foods interact with your child's genetics can impact overall health and ADHD symptoms. The MC4R gene may affect dopamine pathways, appetite regulation, and impulsivity and may increase the risk of ADHD, though the exact link is still under study. Metabolic genes like MC4R also interact with circadian rhythm genes (covered in Step Three – Sleep), further complicating the picture.

SNP Peek - Metabolic Genes

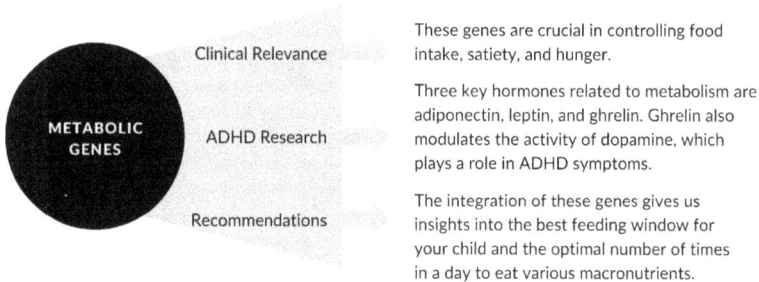

METABOLIC GENES

Clinical Relevance — These genes are crucial in controlling food intake, satiety, and hunger.

ADHD Research — Three key hormones related to metabolism are adiponectin, leptin, and ghrelin. Ghrelin also modulates the activity of dopamine, which plays a role in ADHD symptoms.

Recommendations — The integration of these genes gives us insights into the best feeding window for your child and the optimal number of times in a day to eat various macronutrients.

Other metabolic genes, such as **ADIPOQ, ADRB2, PPARg**, and **FTO**, impact three hormones—adiponectin, leptin, and ghrelin—that regulate appetite, energy balance, and metabolism.

- Adiponectin has anti-inflammatory effects and influences cognitive function, mood, and ADHD symptoms.

- Leptin regulates satiety and impacts reward processing and impulse control, challenges central to ADHD.

- Ghrelin, the "hunger hormone," stimulates appetite and may contribute to impulsive eating, neurodevelopment, and neuroprotection.

The integration of these genes can give insights into your child's feeding window (i.e., times in the day to start and finish eating) and an optimal number of times a day for eating—food in general—and starchier carbohydrates specifically. While all children would do well to eat at least three times a day, with one-third of each of their protein, carbohydrate, and fat intake at each feeding time, some may do better eating about an hour after getting up. Others may feel hungry and ready for food 90-120 minutes after waking.

Because children's stomachs are smaller than those of adults, they may need an afterschool or post-supper snack. Generally, however, if children are getting enough of the right types of nutrients at their primary meals, four or five daily periods of re-fueling, leaving at least two hours between each meal or snack, should be enough.

If your child constantly says they are hungry or hides sweets in their room for snacks, they may need to eat more or get additional protein or fat in their food intake. Rather than relying on these longer-burning fuels, their body is looking to quick-action sugar or ultra-processed foods for energy.

While carbohydrates are crucial in fueling a child, getting the right amount goes a long way toward balancing blood sugar levels and helping your child better cope with challenging situations.

Looking ahead to Step Six – Inflammation, where we discuss the many contributing factors to inflammation, including what we eat, note that adiponectin, leptin, and ghrelin also play a role in inflammation.

Macronutrients

Most of us are aware of the importance of macronutrients—carbohydrates, proteins, and fats—especially in managing ADHD. Let's unpack the genetics behind them.

SNP Peek - Macronutrient Genes

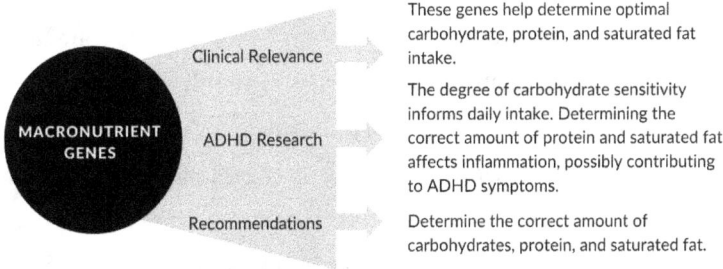

MACRONUTRIENT GENES

Clinical Relevance → These genes help determine optimal carbohydrate, protein, and saturated fat intake.

ADHD Research → The degree of carbohydrate sensitivity informs daily intake. Determining the correct amount of protein and saturated fat affects inflammation, possibly contributing to ADHD symptoms.

Recommendations → Determine the correct amount of carbohydrates, protein, and saturated fat.

Carbohydrates

First, let's differentiate between simple and complex carbohydrates. Simple carbohydrates include sugars and starches in starchy vegetables like potatoes and grains like wheat and rice. Complex carbohydrates, like those in fruits and vegetables, take longer to break down and provide fiber to support gut health.

Most of us love carbohydrates—potato chips, bread, pasta. However, genetic variations in genes like **GIPR**, **TCF7L2**, and **IRS1** may influence the amount your child can tolerate. These SNPs provide insights into factors such as your body's insulin response to carbohydrates, blood sugar stability, and the potential for inflammatory responses in the gastrointestinal tract following carbohydrate consumption.

I (Alicia) remember that at one point, the size of the bags of potato chips available in Mexican school cafeterias was decreased, with the idea being to reduce students' intake of potato chips by selling only the smaller bags of chips. Not only did their experiment fail—students simply purchased multiple smaller bags—since the most expensive part of a bag of chips is the wrapping, the new practice greatly benefited the food industry. Students ate more chips, the increased number of bags contributed to more garbage, and the potato chip companies reaped more profit.

Why do I tell you this story? Because most of us love potato chips. Later, you will be introduced to our concept of Sometimes Food and why you may want to add potato chips to that category.

If you notice your child's relationship with simple carbohydrates seems problematic (e.g., hyperactivity after eating a lot of sugar or starchy carbohydrates, seeming obsession or addiction to sugary or high-carbohydrate-content foods), note that simple carbohydrates rapidly convert to simple sugars, and it may be that their intake of simple carbohydrates is too much for them.

Several studies suggest that diet, particularly sugar intake, may play a role in the development or exacerbation of ADHD symptoms. One reason is that sugar triggers a dopamine release in the brain. Dopamine is part of our brain's natural reward system because eating, particularly foods with a quick energy release, is seen as beneficial for survival.

Because sugar prompts a quick and robust dopamine release, it can lead to cravings and overconsumption as the body adapts to the dopamine response—a dampening of the dopamine receptors, as it were—and requires a higher sugar intake to get a similar reaction. Sugar-seeking behavior can almost be ensured, with potentially volatile reactions, when it is initially withheld.

Consider how your child reacts after eating a large serving of simple carbohydrates. If they are particularly sensitive to carbohydrates (heterozygous or homozygous for variant in the carbohydrate genes mentioned), their blood sugar levels may elevate quickly and come down quickly. When blood sugar is high, you may find some hyperactivity, whereas when it comes down, there might be tantrums or frustration responses.

These genes offer clues about carbohydrate intake: Everyone needs a daily intake of low-starch vegetables (complex carbohydrates), but, depending upon genetics, starchier foods (e.g., rice, grains, fruit, legumes, and sweet potatoes) should be eaten at one, two, or all three meals a day. However, the amount of that simple carbohydrate will range from half to two-thirds the physical size of the protein eaten at the meal.

In North America, it's common for simple carbohydrates to make up half or more of the contents of a meal. That means that no matter what your child's genetic makeup, it's likely that our recommendations will be less bread, pasta, cereal, and muffins and more cucumbers with trail mix, scrambled eggs with peppers, nut butter with celery, and carrot sticks and meatballs than they are accustomed to eating.

Complex carbohydrates include substances like cellulose, hemicellulose, and pectin. They are present in plant cells and are found in fruits and vegetables. Complex carbohydrates take longer to break down, and some are never broken down at all. However, they provide food for our normal flora and play a role in a healthy gut microbiome. They also bring a lot of natural color to our plates!

In simple terms, we call these complex carbohydrates fiber and consider them material that may benefit our intestines. Regular bowel movements are essential for everyone, especially for your child with ADHD. Without sufficient fiber, bowel movements can be sporadic, which only promotes more toxicity in the body (more on this in Step Four - Detox).

As already mentioned, remember to model your vegetable intake for your child. This is a primary reason—along with developing good communication and bonding—we advocate family meal times. Show your child the beautiful, colorful plate you have in front of you, and then have them watch you munch all those tasty vegetables.

A final point here re: vegetable intake and a child not keen on vegetables. Note that your child will eat when they are hungry, and in following Ellyn Satter's division of responsibility, your role is to:

- Choose and prepare the food (which we suggest includes vegetables of some type)

- Provide regular meals and snacks (which we suggest consist of real food)

- Not give your child food or beverages, other than water, between meals and snacks

I (Alicia) remember a phone conversation I had with a mom. She told me her son hadn't had a vegetable in weeks. I simply told her he would eat some when hungry, especially when there was nothing else to nibble on. After about 15 minutes, I heard the child's voice saying: *"Can I finish it?"* The mom gave him some cucumber while we chatted, and he happily finished the snack. She was surprised that a shift could be as simple as that.

Another suggestion is to avoid keeping ultra-processed food in your home. That way, your child is more likely to find something nutritious to enjoy. Make the foods that best support health highly available (e.g., if they open the fridge at a designated snack time, there are washed and cut-up vegetables that are easy to grab and snack on).

When my (Alicia) kids were younger, the easiest way to give them vegetables was before dinner. They would come into the kitchen and tell me they were hungry. Since the only thing on the table was veggies, I told them they could start with what was on the table. Usually, once we sat together for dinner, they had already finished their vegetable intake for the meal!

Also, remember that, for your budget, the most cost-effective way to eat a meal or snack is to start with low-starch vegetables, which almost everyone, regardless of genetics, can tolerate.

Protein

Most of us are aware that protein-rich foods include plant sources like beans, nuts, and seeds or animal sources like beef, pork, chicken, lamb, bison, fish, eggs, or dairy. However, the role of protein's building blocks, amino acids, is not always as well understood. Amino acids have many functions in the body but, in particular, play a role in hormone production. Protein intake, therefore, is essential for anyone, but especially for someone with ADHD.

We look at the **FTO** gene for clues on the optimal amount of protein we need daily (e.g., depending upon whether one is green, yellow, or red in their coding, 0.6 to 1.2 g per kg of body weight). The FTO gene is also known for regulating body weight and fat mass and is strongly associated with obesity. Emerging research suggests that this gene may also be linked to ADHD, mainly through its influence on neural pathways that regulate reward processing, appetite, and impulsivity.

Some studies have found that specific FTO genotypes are associated with lower dopamine D2 receptor availability (more on this gene in Step Five – Calm), which, in turn, is related to cognitive function and reward processing. This suggests that FTO may influence behaviors related to dopamine signaling, such as impulsivity and reward sensitivity, which are relevant to conditions like obesity and possibly ADHD.

Next, let's cover amino acids found in proteins, like L-tyrosine and tryptophan. These serve as building blocks for neurotransmitters like dopamine and serotonin, which play crucial roles in attention and mood regulation. The FTO gene offers excellent insight into the daily amount of protein your child should consume. Those that are homozygous for normal need the least amount of protein, roughly 0.6 to 0.8 g per kg (or 2.2 pounds) of body weight per day. Those that are homozygous for the variant need the most protein per day, approximately

1 to 1.2 g per kg of body weight per day. Those heterozygous require somewhere mid-range, 0.8 to 1 g per kg of body weight daily.

Up to 5 more grams of protein may be required at each of three meals during growth spurts or when children are particularly active in sports or other strenuous activities.

If your child is not consuming enough protein throughout the day to be appropriately supplied with these amino acids, challenges with self-regulation or focus can be exacerbated.

Fats

Our nervous system—and 60% of the brain—is made of fat. So, paying attention to fat intake is essential for optimal brain function.

Let's start by checking several genes that give clues as to the amount of saturated fat—typically solid at room temperature like butter, coconut oil, chicken skin, and found in dairy products—we should consume daily. These genes are **FABP2**, our previously mentioned FTO, and **APOA2**.

If we think about APOA2 as a marker of saturated fat, there aren't conclusive studies on its relationship with ADHD. APOA2 is an indicator of lipid metabolism, and as mentioned before, lipids or fats are essential for the brain to function correctly. However, there is evidence that diets high in saturated fats are associated with cognitive deficits and behavioral issues, including increased inattention and hyperactivity, which are core symptoms of ADHD.

So, on the one hand, we need sufficient saturated fat to provide the raw materials for optimal brain and neuron functioning. On the other hand, we want to ensure that saturated fat intake is not so high that it contributes, through factors such as increased inflammation, to the issues we seek to alleviate. In our practices, we have noticed decreased overall inflammation when one can optimize saturated fat intake based on genetics.

Is there a Goldilocks amount of saturated fat intake for your child? Rather than eating too much or severely restricting saturated fat, could our genetic makeup give us clues on optimizing daily saturated fat intake? The answer is yes.

The clues the APOA2 gene provides regarding how much daily saturated fat someone should consume are very helpful. We primarily use the APOA2 gene to determine the daily amount of saturated fat with a daily intake range between 22 g and 40 g, depending upon genotype, as the norm. For those homozygous for the variant, 22 g daily would be a helpful amount of saturated fat to aim for; for those who are heterozygous (one normal and one variant allele), 28 g daily would be a good amount to target; and for those homozygous for normal, 30-40 g daily would be more appropriate.

Keep in mind that you will need to divide your child's daily intake of saturated fat between their three meals (or three meals and a snack or two); don't have them attempt to eat that allotment all at once!

One final point to add about saturated fat (and for many, it is good news!) is that dark chocolate contains saturated fat. If you are sugar-tolerant (can do a little sugar without that sugar triggering a binge or addictive tendencies), and can handle a little caffeine, if you didn't get your daily saturated fat intake, a square of dark chocolate can often make up the deficit. I (Alicia) have one small square of dark chocolate after lunch and dinner. When I grew up, it seemed that you didn't finish a meal without dessert, so a square of dark chocolate has taken over that role. Once I have that, I don't feel the need to eat anything else until my next scheduled meal. If that sounds like it would work for you, try it!

Along with saturated fat intake, we also need to consider unsaturated fat intake, found in olives, avocados, olive oil, and avocado oil, as well as omega-3 and omega-6 fatty acids, for example, which play a crucial role in brain health and cognitive function. Studies have shown that deficiencies in these essential fatty acids—essential, meaning our diet must supply it as our body can't make it—may contribute to the development or exacerbation of ADHD symptoms. Omega-3 fatty acids, found in high concentrations in the brain, are essential for maintaining neuronal function and reducing inflammation. Several studies suggest that supplementation with omega-3s can improve attention, reduce hyperactivity, and support overall cognitive function in individuals with ADHD. Conversely, diets lacking in these healthy fats may lead to the worsening of ADHD symptoms.

Micronutrients

This book won't cover micronutrients in-depth, but it's important to note that they often act as cofactors with amino acids in proteins, helping them function optimally.

While micronutrients (vitamins and minerals needed in small amounts) are crucial for overall health, we don't typically recommend starting with a multivitamin. Most high-quality multivitamins—primarily due to them containing B2, B6, B12 and folate— support a cellular process called methylation, which can lead to inflammation, especially if detoxification isn't functioning optimally. For many children, reducing inflammation is vital in alleviating some ADHD symptoms. So, we suggest lowering inflammation and improving detoxification pathways (more on this in Step Four – Detox) before introducing a high-quality multivitamin where the vitamins and minerals are in forms best absorbed by the body (e.g., chelated).

A few key micronutrients should be considered.

Zinc is essential for brain function, and deficiencies are linked to increased ADHD symptoms. Dr. Greenblatt has highlighted zinc's importance, noting that copper pipes in homes often result in a zinc-copper imbalance, disrupting neurotransmitter balance. Adding zinc to the diet or through a highly absorbable supplement (i.e., zinc glycinate) may help reduce ADHD symptoms. Dr. Greenblatt shared a story about an orange orchard where the trees started producing fruit after zinc-containing nails were used to post For Sale signs, illustrating zinc's impact on growth and productivity (and may have meant the orchard no longer needed to be sold!).

Magnesium, the "relaxation mineral," is a micronutrient we often recommend for children with ADHD. When choosing the best form of magnesium for your child, it's important to consider the specific benefits you're hoping to achieve. Each form of magnesium offers unique advantages, so understanding these can help you make an informed decision.

- **Cognitive Functioning:** Magnesium L-threonate is a particularly effective form of magnesium supplementation for ADHD. Its unique ability to cross the blood-brain barrier enhances magnesium levels in the brain, which are crucial for cognitive functions such as attention, memory, and learning—areas often impacted in individuals with ADHD.

- **Digestion/Constipation:** Magnesium Citrate is another form with high bioavailability, meaning it's well-absorbed by the body. It's commonly used to support muscle and nerve function and alleviate constipation. While its role in nerve health may offer some benefits for ADHD, its primary applications are related to digestive support and muscle function.

- **Calming/Mood:** Magnesium Glycinate is known for its calming effects and is often recommended to support mood and relaxation. While it may reduce anxiety and improve sleep quality, which can be beneficial for individuals with ADHD, it doesn't specifically target cognitive functions as effectively as Magnesium L-threonate.

While zinc and magnesium are good examples, we also recommend ensuring an adequate intake of other essential micronutrients, such as vitamins B6, B12, D, and folate. Vitamin D supports mood and cognitive function, while B6 is crucial for neurotransmitter production.

Methylation is a biochemical process in which a methyl group (one carbon atom and three hydrogen atoms) is added to molecules. It plays a critical role in DNA repair, detoxification, and neurotransmitter production (a good thing!). However, if inflammation is unresolved, introducing methylation support too early can overstimulate pathways, potentially worsening symptoms instead of restoring balance (not good!).

While nutrients like zinc, magnesium, and vitamin D influence methylation indirectly, they do not donate a methyl group. These nutrients carry minimal risk of overstimulating methylation and provide additional benefits, making them generally safe to start anytime. In contrast, some B vitamins (B2, B6, B12) and folate directly affect methylation pathways, so addressing and reducing inflammation before introducing these supplements is important.

Lastly, probiotics, beneficial bacteria for gut health, are also worth considering. Research suggests a healthy gut microbiome can positively affect brain function and behavior. Start by incorporating probiotic-rich fermented foods like sauerkraut, pickles, kimchi, and quality, low-sugar content yogurt into your family's diet. And, if need be, when choosing a probiotic, ensure it is from human strains, has been highly researched and tested, and contains the amount your child needs to see an impact on their health. Genestra's HMF line follows that criteria and contains specific strains to support cognitive function and address gut-brain issues.

Personalizing Nutrition per Genetics

Imagine fueling a high-performance sports car with regular gasoline—it might run, but not at its best. Similarly, your child's brain needs the right balance of macronutrients to function optimally. Personalized nutrition, or metabolic typing, is a fascinating science we've used in our practices for decades.

The bottom line? Due to genetic variations, different bodies require different amounts of protein, fats, and carbohydrates. For example, variations in the FTO gene impact how the body processes fats and sugars, and, as mentioned, this gene also gives clues about protein needs. These genetic variations can influence how an individual responds to their diet, affecting behavior and health outcomes. Understanding such differences is crucial for tailoring nutritional approaches to better suit your child's unique needs.

Macronutrients—proteins, fats, and carbohydrates—each play a unique role in supporting brain function and overall health. Protein helps produce neurotransmitters like dopamine and serotonin, essential for mood regulation and focus. Healthy sources include meats, fish, poultry, beans, and tofu. Carbohydrates provide energy, but complex carbs (whole grains, vegetables, fruit) offer a steady supply without the crashes caused by simple sugars. Fats, especially omega-3s found in salmon, walnuts, and flaxseeds, are vital for brain health.

Watch for signs that your child might be getting too much or too little of a macronutrient. Constant hunger or energy crashes could indicate too many carbohydrates, while frequent fatigue might signal that your child needs more protein or fat.

The goal is to find the right fuel mix for your child's genetic makeup. Operate with trial and error until you find the correct ratio or access our free children's Dietary Needs Assessment, "What Veggie Are You?" This tool, found in our *Kids Activity Book* (free download here: https://www.inbalancelm.com/ADHD_kid sbook-triplog), helps determine whether your child is a Protein (Snappy), Carbohydrate (Carrot Top) or Mixed Body Type (Buddy). Once you identify your child's type, the activity book gives personalized dietary and lifestyle tips.

TRAVELER ASSISTANCE

Easy Steps to Get Started with a Food Plan

If you've decided not to pursue DNA testing at this time, start with what we've done with clients for decades.

Begin with In BALANCE Principles

The In BALANCE (IB) pyramid was created to simplify nutritional and lifestyle planning. At its foundation, you'll find the acronym BALANCE: B for Body Type, A for Attitude, L for Laughter and Play, A for Activity, N for a good Night's Sleep, C for Clean Water, and E for Eat for Health. That base provides the essentials for overall well-being. Moving up, you'll see the macronutrients—proteins, fats, and carbohydrates—adjusted to individual needs. And yes, there's a place for Sometimes Food because celebration is essential too.

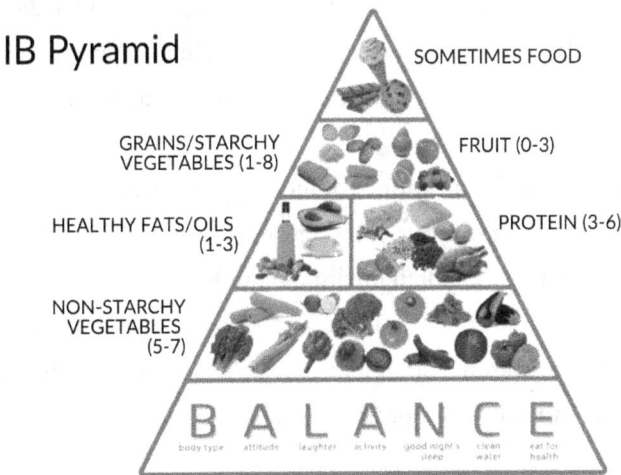

IB Pyramid

SOMETIMES FOOD

GRAINS/STARCHY VEGETABLES (1-8)

FRUIT (0-3)

HEALTHY FATS/OILS (1-3)

PROTEIN (3-6)

NON-STARCHY VEGETABLES (5-7)

B A L A N C E

body type   attitude   laughter   activity   good night's sleep   clean water   eat for health

Dietary Plans

The Mediterranean diet is often recommended for its brain-boosting benefits. Rich in fruits, vegetables, whole grains, and healthy fats, this diet supports brain health and can help reduce ADHD symptoms. Eating a diet low in processed foods and high in nutrient-dense options is ideal. Feeding windows, with set times for meals and snacks, can help regulate blood sugar and reduce impulsivity, another good strategy for ADHD.

Elimination Diets

Elimination diets can also be effective. You can see if symptoms improve by removing potential allergens like artificial colors, preservatives, and certain food groups. Up to 30% of children with ADHD may benefit from elimination diets, notably removing dyes, gluten, or dairy. The success of these diets often depends on your child's detoxification genes, which affect how efficiently their body processes and eliminates substances.

Meal Planning

Planning ADHD-friendly meals can feel overwhelming, but you don't need to overcomplicate it! Start with a weekly plan that includes a variety of whole foods—fresh fruit, vegetables, lean proteins, and whole grains. Meal prepping (e.g., bulk cooking or chopping vegetables ahead of time) and delegating tasks to all family members can be a lifesaver for busy families. Prepare ingredients in advance to make meals quick and easy. Remember that different family members might need tailored portions based on their unique macronutrient needs.

Sometimes Food

Sometimes, food may be less nutritious or more expensive, but they bring joy and celebration. Depending on your child's genetics, their tolerance for these foods may vary. For example, children predisposed to higher inflammation may need to limit sugar and refined grains more strictly. Instead, their "Sometimes Food" may be an out-of-season fruit or a fun (more expensive, thus the "sometimes") protein such as a lamb chop or sirloin steak.

Supplements

Supplements can help fill nutritional gaps, but should always *supplement* a healthy diet. While we'll cover more specific supplements in future Steps, consider high-quality, whole-food options like plant-based gummies or moringa powder for this Step. Supplements can support overall health, especially when certain nutrients are challenging to get from food alone.

REST STOP

It's time for parents to take a break and digest information! Take 10 minutes of calm to Rest with the following questions:

1. **Your Relationship With Food:** As parents are generally the primary shoppers and meal preppers in a household, how has your relationship with food impacted the types and varieties of food available in your home? Can you see where examining some of the reasoning for certain choices (e.g., ultra-processed food amounts, limited fresh produce) could be vital in moving forward?

2. **Moving Toward Wellness:** Would you consider changing some of your purchases from ones that no longer serve you or your child well to choices that better support overall household wellness?

Next, Stop for 10 minutes of quiet (sitting or slowly walking). Keep your mind as clear and open as possible, and just listen. Jot down or tell Siri to "make a note" of any responses that may arise. Because you've taken time to ponder calmly and quietly, these responses will most likely be less off-the-cuff and from a deeper level. They can give you clues as to the reasons behind your answers! Those clues, in turn, will reveal potential problematic thinking and can provide great direction on moving forward with the recommendations in this Step that would be the easiest to implement or fit best for your family!

ROADWORK

Food and Mood Tracker

Materials:

- A notebook or digital device

- Pen

Directions:

1. **Divide Your Page:** Create sections for different meals and snacks

throughout the day.

2. **Log Your Meals:** Write down what your child eats at each meal and snack.

3. **Note the Mood:** Observe and note any changes in your child's behavior or mood before and after eating.

4. **Identify Patterns:** At the end of the week, review the journal to identify any patterns or correlations between food and mood.

When you do the Food/Mood log with your children, you will be able to note changes that occur as you incorporate new foods, potentially adjust your child's feeding window, and optimize your child's intake of macronutrients. Have conversations with your child about any changes made and results experienced so they can grow in listening to their body.

Potential changes to watch for are:

- Is your child bloated?

- Does your child have increased or decreased physical energy?

- Is your child more or less mentally alert?

- What is your child's mood after a specific meal or food intake?

This simple activity helps you understand how different foods affect your child's behavior and mood, making it easier to tailor their diet to their needs.

As a final note on this activity, why not complete a Food and Mood Tracker for yourself as well? You will not only be modeling the use of a helpful tool for your child but may also discover some very interesting links for yourself!

SOUVENIR

For this Step's souvenirs, we'd like you to ensure your child is getting enough water and come up with great lunch ideas!

There isn't a "water intake" gene, but hydration is key for everyone. So, we encourage you and your child to keep track of it and notice any changes in behavior during the day when keeping hydrated.

We are constantly asked about Menu planning. I (Alicia) am the type of person who gets into the kitchen, opens the fridge, and mixes things randomly when I cook. Brenda, on the other hand, likes a more structured cooking approach, with meal planning and recipes.

Thus, we created *"Lickety-Split Lunches"* and included them in the *Kids Activity Book*. With this easy infographic, highlights of which you'll find here, your child will understand the ratio of macronutrients their body needs, per the *What Veggie Are You* survey, and how to mix and match them depending on their body type. Working together to prepare meals is an excellent way to get your child involved in food prep, and you can have a great time connecting with them in the best place in the house: the kitchen!

BUDDY SQUASH
Mixed Body Type

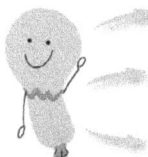

Can have more variety in food choices and include options from both carbohydrate (Carrot Top) and protein (Snappy) body type fuel mix.

Should eat relatively equal ratios of proteins/fats and grains/vegetables. That means a fuel mix of 40-50% protein-rich foods and fat and 50-60% veggies, safe starches, and fruit.

In order to feel most energized and maintain ideal weight may need to adjust either the percentage of carbohydrate-rich foods or fat servings.

2 servings protein
1-2 servings carbohydrates
3-4 servings vegetables
1/2 - 1 serving fat
1-2 servings fruit

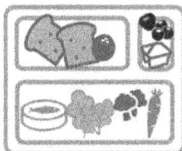

SNAPPY
Protein Body Type

Needs regular intake of the proteins found in red meats and oily fish like salmon.

Limits intake of whole grains and starchy vegetables like potatoes.

Eats lots of food from the non-starchy vegetables category like spinach, bell peppers, and asparagus.

Limits fruit intake to a maximum of 1 piece per day, choosing low-sugar options like apples, dark berries, and grapefruit.

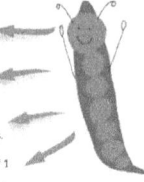

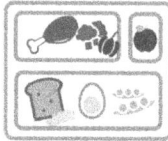

2 servings protein
1 serving carbohydrates
3 servings vegetables
1-2 servings fat
1 serving fruit

CARROT TOP
Carbohydrate Body Type

Focuses protein intake on lighter options such as white meats, legumes, nuts, and seeds.

Eats moderate amounts of sprouted whole grain bread, brown rice, and other whole grains and starchy vegetables.

May consume 2-3 servings of fruit per day; choose whole fruits over juices!

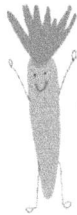

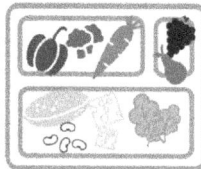

2 servings protein
2 servings carbohydrates
4 servings vegetables
1/2 serving fat
1-2 servings fruit

And if your child with ADHD is a pre-teen or adolescent, then, instead, do the following activity with them.

Food Scrabble

This simple game can help family members think of new food items to try in the In BALANCE Pyramid food groups.

Materials:

- Pens or pencils

- Paper

- One six-sided die

- Scrabble tiles or all the letters of the alphabet, individually printed on equal-sized cards or pieces of paper

- A chalkboard or large piece of paper taped to a wall, door, or window

Directions:
- On a chalkboard or large piece of paper, write: 1=Non Starchy Vegetables; 2=Protein; 3=Healthy Fats and Oils; 4=Fruits; 5=Grains and Starchy Vegetables; 6=Sometimes Foods.

- Take turns rolling the dice and randomly choosing a letter.

- Participants then have 30 seconds to write down as many names as possible of foods that start with the letter they picked from the category corresponding to the number of their dice roll.

- Whoever comes up with the most words in each round scores a point.

- Continue playing to a set number of points (5 or 10).

Tips:
- You may need to adjust the time limit depending on the participants' ages and levels of writing ability (e.g., allow younger family members 30-60 seconds more per turn).

- For a larger group, separate the participants into two teams and have teams come up with answers together.

- Omit letters such as X and Q or allow them to be used in an item name instead of having to start a name.

Now, let's explore how movement and exercise play a role in managing ADHD symptoms.

Chapter 5

Core Step Two - Move

"Exercise turns on the attention system, the so-called executive functions — sequencing, working memory, prioritizing, inhibiting, and sustaining attention. On a practical level, it causes kids to be less impulsive, which makes them more primed to learn."
- Dr. John Ratey, author of Spark: The Revolutionary New Science
of Exercise and the Brain

SUMMARY - Travel Size Version

It's a rainy Saturday afternoon, and you're at an indoor gym watching your child race around the play area. They swing from the climbing apparatus, chase friends, and suddenly stop to examine an abandoned set of building blocks. Sitting on the bench, you wonder how all this energy can be channeled to help manage ADHD symptoms. At least part of the answer is understanding how physical activity can naturally support challenging ADHD behaviors.

Movement's Role in Managing ADHD

We'll start with some science on how physical activity enhances brain development and neurobehavioral functioning, focusing on three key genes. Regular physical activity helps regulate brain chemicals like dopamine and norepinephrine, which are essential for focus and self-control.

Joyful Movement

Understanding the benefits of physical activity for ADHD is one thing, but it's just as crucial for your child to find movement they enjoy. Think about what they love ... we'll start there!

Simple Ways to Incorporate Movement in Your Family

Knowing why movement is essential and what your child enjoys is excellent, but setting that plan into action can be challenging. Here, we'll get creative with ways to fit more movement into your daily schedule.

Supplements that Support Healthy Movement

We'll also explore supplements that could support your child's exercise habits, depending on their genetics.

As Nike says, "Just Do It."

To make movement more engaging, we'll provide instructions for creating a movement chart for your child to track activities.

INFORMATION CENTER

Physical Activity as a Natural Therapy for ADHD

There is convincing evidence that physical exercise enhances brain development and neurobehavioral functioning in areas of potential impairment in children with ADHD. That's one reason a mom we know whose son has ADHD ensures he gets plenty of movement during the day to help him calm down at night. Their family's solution? Her son plays many hours of soccer every single day of the week.

Now, what is the link between different types of exercise, from sprinting to endurance, and its relationship with ADHD? And how can our genes determine which kind of exercise is better for us in terms of the type of fibers we have in our muscles?

Three genes can give us clues as to what type of exercise is best for your child. They are **ACTN3**, **ADRB2**, and **ACE**. The different combinations of these genes shed light on whether we have a lot of fast twitch fibers for sprinting or an abundance of slow twitch fibers that are effective for prolonged exercise and, therefore, are designed more for endurance-type exercises. Those genes also help determine if we do better with longer cardiovascular workouts, at a moderate or slower pace, or with a High-Intensity Interval Training (HIIT) activity where our pace is varied between faster activity and slower recovery activity.

Some of the benefits of endurance exercise, such as running, swimming, cycling, or walking, are that it boosts dopamine and norepinephrine levels. Regular aerobic (with oxygen) activity can help by increasing these neurotransmitters in the brain, improving attention, focus, and mood. Endurance exercises can also reduce stress and anxiety (more about this in Step Five – Calm).

High-intensity interval training in sports like basketball, soccer, and hockey, for example, where a player uses bursts of speed, can also lead to a rapid increase of dopamine and norepinephrine levels that, as mentioned earlier, can improve mood and motivation.

So, while both types of activity can enhance dopamine and norepinephrine production, comparing sprinting to endurance has found that sprinting provides more immediate, short-term benefits for focus and energy levels, whereas endurance exercise results in long-term benefits.

SNP Peek - Move Genes

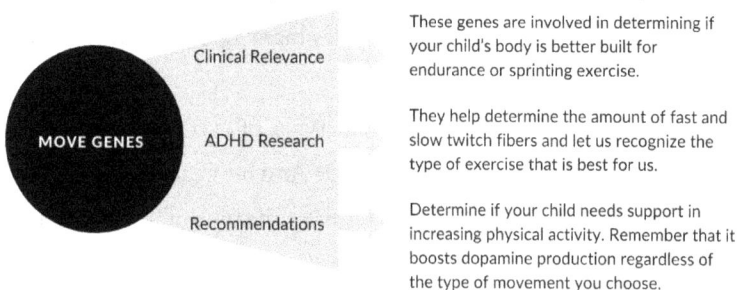

MOVE GENES

Clinical Relevance

ADHD Research

Recommendations

These genes are involved in determining if your child's body is better built for endurance or sprinting exercise.

They help determine the amount of fast and slow twitch fibers and let us recognize the type of exercise that is best for us.

Determine if your child needs support in increasing physical activity. Remember that it boosts dopamine production regardless of the type of movement you choose.

Finding Joy in Movement

Besides the neurotransmitter aspect, different types of exercise can offer a wide variety of benefits for a child with ADHD. However, finding activities that resonate with your child's interests and genetic predispositions is essential.

I (Alicia) grew up in a highly academic family where exercise was not the focus. It was not until recently that I found my love for walking. The day I don't do it, I truly miss it! We encourage you to find that type of exercise—even if it means you have a bit of trial and error— where your child loves it so much that they will miss it and want more.

If your child is willing to try team sports, for example, they provide an excellent opportunity for children with ADHD to develop social skills, learn teamwork, and burn off excess energy. Sports like flag football, lacrosse, or volleyball can be great options.

Martial arts, such as karate or taekwondo, are also highly beneficial. They require focus, discipline, and coordination, which can help improve attention and impulse control. Additionally, non-group activities like swimming, track, fencing, and dance can be more suitable for some children. They offer a structured yet enjoyable way to stay active without the pressure of team competition.

Whatever type of exercise your child with ADHD does, you can be assured that it will help them be calmer and happier. So, the best plan is to have them discover a movement that brings them joy.

For that, you'll want to:

Expose them to a range of activities at a reasonably early age. On family outings, try hiking, swimming, biking, or climbing different types of playground apparatus. Perhaps do as we did in my (Brenda's) family and have them register for a different activity each season.

Over the years, we covered the spectrum from soccer to rugby to basketball to skiing to baseball, to water polo to handball to ballet to volleyball to snowboarding to ball hockey to football to swimming and diving to breakdancing to skateboarding. Sometimes, the activity wasn't particularly enjoyable (e.g., baseball, ballet), and our child only did it for one season. Some activities became favorite movements and continued into adulthood (e.g., soccer, snowboarding, mountain biking, volleyball).

Recognize your child's unique emotional and physical affinity for an activity. We've looked at muscle fiber as a clue. While other genes may influence muscle soreness or injury susceptibility, affecting which activities suit your child best (and, incidentally, how often you need to replace their sports shoes and the amount of K-tape you purchase), here we're focused on emotional preferences for different types of activity. Some children with ADHD enjoy playing and doing activities with others. They can do quite well with social engagement once they eat, move, sleep, and supplement to minimize situational mismatches. They like team sports and the camaraderie that can occur in that environment.

Other children prefer to do activities that involve less interaction with others. They find swimming lengths to be enjoyable and calming. Solo runs—or running with a partner they don't necessarily need to talk with—are more their fit. Take time to observe and dialogue with your child about the different types of activities they are engaged in. Ask how a particular kind of movement feels in your child's "brain" or analytical thinking part of themselves. Then, ask how the activity feels in their "heart" or feeling part of themselves. They may initially feel nervous and a bit afraid brain-wise to try or stick with an activity, but when they check in with their heart, they realize a part of them wants to give it a try for at least a while longer.

Simple Ways to Make Movement Work

Incorporating more physical activity into your child's daily routine doesn't have to be a Herculean task. If registering for a season-long sport seems daunting, start with small, manageable changes, like drop-in gym sessions, that fit your family's schedule. The key is finding activities everyone enjoys, making it easier to stick to a routine. For example, you could take a brisk walk together after dinner, turn weekend errands into a family bike ride, or play a quick game of tag in the backyard.

I (Alicia) remember when my kids were younger, and we walked after dinner; our time included a lot of chatting. One day, when we walked around a long block, I told my two daughters it was time to head back home. The younger one said: "But I haven't talked yet!" Her older sister had been the primary one chatting with me. So, we happily went around the block twice to give the youngest a chance to share what was on her mind as well. I realized then that walking is one of the best things to do when you want to talk with your child, especially if they are not keen on participating in that chat. Something about the fact that you are not directly looking into their eyes but are walking alongside them seems to encourage conversation. Bottom line? Walk with your kids. The entire family can benefit from movement anyway, and you might have excellent communication along the way.

For those days when time is tight, perhaps even too tight for a short walk, even something as simple as skipping for one minute can increase dopamine production and provide a quick energy boost. The goal is to make physical activity a regular part of your child's life and provide a tool to help them regulate some of ADHD's more challenging symptoms naturally and effectively.

Max, a ten-year-old boy diagnosed with ADHD, struggled with staying focused in school and often acted out in class. His parents decided to enroll him in a local basketball league, hoping the physical activity would help channel his energy. After a few months, Max's teachers noticed significant improvements in his behavior and focus. The structured environment of the basketball team, combined with the physical exertion, helped Max manage his symptoms better. On the other hand, Lily is an eight-year-old girl who found absolute joy in developing a martial art. The discipline and focus required in her karate classes helped her learn to control her impulses and improve her concentration.

Movement should definitely be an essential part of your child's day to help them see helpful changes in their dopamine levels. It can also help them achieve positive results, such as calmness and better managing challenging situations. It is up to you and your child to determine what that movement looks like.

A Couple of Additional Notes on Movement

First, we suggest keeping movement earlier in the day, or at least not doing heavy exercise right before bedtime, as it can negatively impact some children's sleep. Secondly, our emphasis on the type of muscle and different forms of movement your child might be best suited to isn't about turning your child into an Olympic athlete—although it appears the prevalence of ADHD among elite athletes is higher than in the general population—but about finding enjoyable, success-enhancing, and muscle type-supporting ways to incorporate movement into their daily routine.

If you and your child can determine the types of activity that cover all those bases, you'll be well on your way to reaping many movement rewards.

I (Brenda) and my husband, Mark, had been athletic as youngsters and adults, and we passed that love of sports on to all five of our children. Rachel wasn't diagnosed with ADHD until her childhood and teenage years were over, but in hindsight, we can see how much benefit she experienced by being constantly involved in sports. Though the family budget meant our kids could only be involved in one sport at a time, all five were involved in one sport or another all year. Rachel was no exception.

She played soccer, basketball, and volleyball and took swimming lessons, honing her focusing skills (as she was in sports she enjoyed) and growing in teamwork and leadership. Rachel's athletic endeavors helped with restlessness, made her physically tired enough to sleep better, and fostered confidence. With the classic 20/20 vision that hindsight allows, we see how regular exercise significantly helped manage her ADHD symptoms. She continues her gym workouts and team sports, even adding new activities like surfing to her routine.

Supplements that Support Healthy Movement

Supplements that support physical activity can also play a role in managing ADHD symptoms. For instance, collagen supplements can help support joint health and muscle recovery, making it easier for your child to stay active without experiencing discomfort. While we didn't cover injury genes in this book, should you find your child experiencing a number of sports injuries (e.g., sprained joints, stretched ligaments, sore muscles), you may want to consider including a homemade or quality purchased bone broth in their diet as it contains a hearty supply of collagen.

Electrolyte supplements can ensure your child stays hydrated and maintains proper muscle function, especially during intense physical activities. These supplements can provide the additional support needed to keep your child engaged in regular exercise, helping to manage their ADHD symptoms more effectively. However, we suggest you carefully read the "sports drinks" label, as many contain high amounts of sugar. Make sure that the electrolyte drink you choose has no coloring, chemicals, and minimal sugar, or have your child make their sports drink by putting about ½ cup of their favorite unsweetened fruit juice in their water bottle (for some quick sugar supply), along with a pinch of sea salt (to cover some of the needed mineral requirements), and then top up the bottle with water. Their homemade version of a sports drink will do the trick by supporting their physical efforts without the ingredients that can foster challenges for some children with ADHD.

Regular physical activity isn't just about managing ADHD symptoms; it's about creating a foundation for overall well-being. By understanding that exercise impacts factors such as neurotransmitters and sleep and considering your child's unique genetic makeup, you can tailor physical activities to meet their needs. The benefits of exercise extend beyond just managing ADHD symptoms; they contribute to a healthier, happier, and more balanced life for your child.

TRAVELER ASSISTANCE

For this Step's Traveler Assistance, we'll highlight the hidden potential of how an ADHD brain functions regarding physical activity. Children with ADHD often have great energy and a natural curiosity that makes them want to explore and move. This can be a big advantage when it comes to staying active. Their natural inclination to move can be harnessed to help them focus better and manage their symptoms. Active movement helps burn off energy and provides a structured way for them to channel their impulses in a positive direction.

Think about it this way: when your child is engaged in physical activity, they're not just burning calories or strengthening muscles; they're also learning essential skills like discipline, patience, and teamwork. These skills can carry over into other areas of their life, helping them succeed in school and social situations. So, while it might feel like a challenge to keep up with their energy levels, remember that this energy—channeled in helpful directions—can be a powerful tool for helping them thrive.

REST STOP

It's time for parents to take a break and digest information! Take 10 minutes of calm to Rest with the following questions:

1. **Your Relationship with Physical Activity:** How did your experiences with physical activity as a child shape your current attitude toward

movement and exercise? Are there beliefs or habits from your past that might influence how active your household is today, and how might these affect your child's experience with physical activity?

2. **Encouraging vs. Forcing Movement:** Consider the balance between encouraging your child to be active and respecting their natural energy levels or preferences. Are there areas where you may be too forceful or lenient about incorporating physical activity? How might finding a middle ground that honors your child's needs and the benefits of movement change the dynamics around physical activity in your family?

Next, Stop for 10 minutes of quiet (sitting or slowly walking). Keep your mind as clear and open as possible, and just listen. Jot down or tell Siri to "make a note" of any responses that may arise. Because you've taken time to ponder calmly and quietly, these responses will most likely be less off-the-cuff and from a deeper level. They can give you clues as to the reasons behind your answers! Those clues, in turn, will reveal potential problematic thinking and can provide great direction on moving forward with the recommendations in this Step that would be the easiest to implement or fit best for your family!

ROADWORK
Fun Move/Mood Log
Materials:

- A large sheet of paper or a whiteboard

- Colorful markers or stickers

Directions:

1. Create the Chart: Create horizontal rows for each day of the week and vertical columns for Mood Before, Type of Activity, Mood After, and Conclusion.

2. List Activities: Write down your child's physical activities daily and include their mood before and after exercise.

3. Track Conclusions: Have a conversation with your child about the ways you are finding exercise impacts their mood.

4. Celebrate: At the end of the week, celebrate their new understanding with a small reward or a fun family outing.

This activity helps your child see their progress, including regular movement and the links between exercise and mood. Plus, it adds an element of fun and celebration to their efforts.

SOUVENIR

We suggest getting each family member something new for their Step Two – Move souvenir to encourage them to be active. Since every household has a different budget allocation, we'll give you various purchase options!

- A pair of playful (i.e., curly) or bright-colored shoelaces to revitalize a pair of sneakers.

- Reusable water bottles so everyone can stay hydrated while being active.

- An outdoor game the family can enjoy (e.g., bocce, badminton).

- Swim passes to enjoy at a local pool.

- An outing to try a new activity (e.g., snowshoeing, snow or wakeboarding, pickleball).

- A low-cost class trial (e.g., yoga, dance).

- New exercise equipment for the household (e.g., basketball hoop, bikes, hiking backpacks).

Pick something enjoyable that works for your family, or choose another option that better suits your household!

Next, we'll explore how sleep is crucial in managing ADHD and offer more strategies for supporting your child's well-being.

Chapter 6

Core Step Three - Sleep

"Sleep is the golden chain that binds health and our bodies together."

- Thomas Dekker, author of The Gull's Hornbook

SUMMARY - Travel Size Version

It's 10 PM, and you've finished the bedtime routine hours ago. You've read a story, given a glass of water, and tucked your child in, only to hear the pitter-patter of little feet roaming the house minutes later. Despite all efforts, your child can't seem to settle down for the night. If this sounds familiar, you're not alone. Many parents of children with ADHD face nightly battles to achieve restful sleep. But what if we told you that understanding the science behind sleep and its impact on ADHD could be a ticket to better sleep for everyone?

The Relationship between Sleep and ADHD

As usual, we'll start this Step by looking at genes—in this case, two that impact sleep.

Sleep and ADHD are closely linked, and children with ADHD often struggle with falling asleep, waking up frequently, or rising too early. In addition, poor quality sleep can also negatively impact ADHD symptoms. However, by making changes to improve sleep quantity and quality for your child with ADHD, you can bring about positive change that benefits all family members!

Circadian Rhythms and Insomnia

A Sleep Step wouldn't be complete without covering our circadian rhythms' wake/sleep effects.

And, because there are a variety of ways your child with ADHD may have sleep disrupted, we'll explore several different types of insomnia ... and what to do about them!

Sleep Hygiene

One key aspect to focus on with your child is establishing a consistent sleep routine. This means having a regular bedtime and wake-up time, even on weekends. Consistency helps regulate your child's internal clock, making it easier for them to fall asleep and wake up refreshed. Think of it like setting a daily alarm for their body.

Supplements to Support Sound Sleep

We will wrap up this Step with supplements to consider for sleep support for your child.

INFORMATION CENTER

The Relationship Between Sleep, ADHD and Gene Expression

In the various Parenting ADHD children FB groups to which we belong, poor sleep—of children and, therefore, parents—is a never-ending thread. It's not just about the children's sleep but also the disruption it causes for parents and other family members. From kids who struggle with bedtime tasks when their medication wears off or still have too much dopamine in their system to settle to those who wake up during the night or too early in the morning, the resulting meltdowns, angry outbursts, and household disruption are a significant part of life for many families with children with ADHD.

Much of the sleep disruption seen with ADHD can be linked to the complex relationship between sleep, genetics, and circadian rhythms. The **CLOCK** gene, often called the master regulator of circadian rhythms, has been closely studied for its role in ADHD. Circadian rhythms are the body's natural biological clock, governing sleep-wake cycles and numerous other physiological functions.

Circadian rhythms operate on roughly 24-hour cycles and are primarily influenced by external cues like light. When the eyes detect light, they trigger a cascade of signals to the brain's suprachiasmatic nucleus (SCN), the body's master clock. This clock promotes wakefulness and suppresses sleep.

How can you tell when your circadian rhythm is functioning optimally? You'll experience a healthy morning cortisol spike, waking with energy and alertness. Cortisol levels should then gradually decline throughout the day, hitting their lowest point in the evening, making falling and staying asleep easier. When circadian rhythms are misaligned—due to irregular schedules, light exposure at the wrong times, or genetic factors—it can delay sleep onset, fragment sleep cycles, or cause early morning awakenings, all commonly reported in children with ADHD. Exposure to light, especially natural sunlight, triggers the cycle to reset each morning, reinforcing the body's internal clock.

When the circadian rhythm master clock is well-aligned, it supports the synchronization of the body's peripheral clocks, which are found in organs such as the pancreas, liver, muscles, and adipose tissue. This synchronization ensures that processes like blood sugar regulation, detoxification, and hormone production function efficiently.

However, because stress and sleep share overlapping physiological pathways, chronic stress can disrupt circadian rhythms, leading to irregular sleep patterns (another of those correlations between our Core Steps).

Research indicates that children with ADHD often experience disruptions in circadian rhythms, contributing to sleep disorders and a preference for an evening chronotype—a tendency to be more alert and active in the evening than in the morning. This misalignment can lead to poor sleep quality and quantity, exacerbating ADHD symptoms. Genetic factors, such as variations in the CLOCK gene, play a significant role in these disruptions. Changes in this gene have been associated with altered circadian patterns, delayed sleep onset, and increased ADHD-related challenges.

Another critical gene implicated in the sleep-ADHD connection is **CRY1**. Variants in this gene are linked to Delayed Sleep Phase Disorder (DSPD), a condition where falling asleep and waking up at socially conventional times becomes difficult. Children with DSPD often experience insomnia, insufficient sleep, and daytime sleepiness. The combined effects of CLOCK and CRY1 gene variants can significantly delay sleep onset, sometimes by several hours, making it challenging to achieve enough restorative sleep cycles.

Sleep traditionally includes four main stages: awake, light sleep, deep sleep, and rapid eye movement (REM) sleep. Each stage serves vital functions for mental and physical health. For instance:

- **Deep sleep** supports tissue growth and repair, cell regeneration, and growth hormone release.

- **REM sleep** is crucial for memory consolidation, learning, problem-solving, and flushing waste from the brain through the glymphatic system.

To fully benefit from sleep, the body ideally cycles through four to five 90-minute sleep cycles during the night. When sleep onset is delayed, your child may struggle to complete these cycles, notably missing critical REM sleep stages. This can feel like waking to an alarm clock but repeatedly hitting the snooze button, resulting in grogginess and reduced cognitive function the next morning.

Focusing on the quality and quantity of sleep is essential for children with ADHD. Deep and sustained sleep is necessary for the body to perform critical functions, and insufficient sleep deprives the brain and body of the time needed for these processes. Addressing genetic and behavioral sleep challenges can significantly improve your child's overall well-being.

Whenever we think "sleep," what comes to our minds is a woman in one of our online epigenetic programs who felt all she needed was four hours of sleep every night. She believed her inability to sleep longer than that was genetic. "I have been like that since I was a child," she said, "And my mom is the same." After following similar principles to those found in this book, she has "reset" her genes. She can sleep eight hours a night and cannot believe how good she feels.

SNP Peek - Sleep Genes

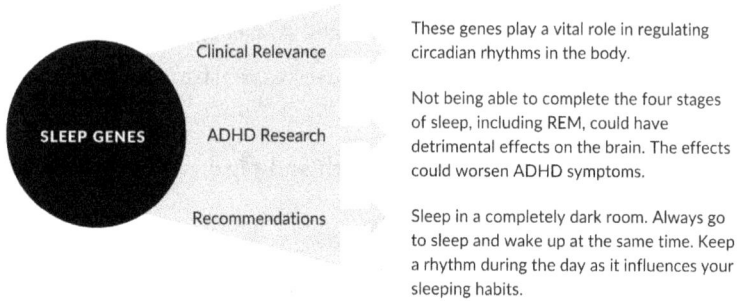

SLEEP GENES

Clinical Relevance

These genes play a vital role in regulating circadian rhythms in the body.

ADHD Research

Not being able to complete the four stages of sleep, including REM, could have detrimental effects on the brain. The effects could worsen ADHD symptoms.

Recommendations

Sleep in a completely dark room. Always go to sleep and wake up at the same time. Keep a rhythm during the day as it influences your sleeping habits.

As reinforcement that the impact of a poor night's sleep is not just felt by children, note that when I (Alicia) don't have a good night's sleep, I wake up grouchy. I don't even want to be with myself! Now that I understand epigenetics, I can see why I was cranky and irritable every morning before I changed my lifestyle and sleep patterns.

While poor sleep has many physiological effects, the bidirectional interaction between sleep and gene expression—each influencing the other—plays a large role in neuroplasticity and neurotransmitter pathway regulation.

Neuroplasticity refers to the brain's ability to reorganize itself by forming new neural connections. This is crucial for learning and memory, areas that already face challenges in ADHD brains. During sleep, especially deep sleep, the brain consolidates memories, clears out toxins, and supports both neuroplasticity and positive gene expression. These restorative processes are essential for maintaining cognitive and emotional health.

Neurotransmitters like dopamine and serotonin, which are critical in ADHD, are also regulated during sleep. This involves maintaining appropriate levels, replenishing reserves, and modulating their release to support balanced brain functioning. Sleep disruption interferes with these pathways, reducing the efficiency of neurotransmitter regulation and altering the brain's reward and emotional regulation systems. When sleep cycles are shortened or disrupted, dopamine and serotonin-dependent processes are impaired, exacerbating ADHD symptoms and making it harder to manage behavior. This creates a vicious cycle, as ADHD symptoms like restlessness and impulsivity can further disrupt sleep, perpetuating the problem.

Circadian Rhythms and Insomnia

As mentioned, circadian rhythms play a significant role in regulating sleep processes. These rhythms, governed by our body's internal clock, influence the timing of various activities such as hormone release, body temperature, and sleep-wake cycles.

Circadian Rhythm

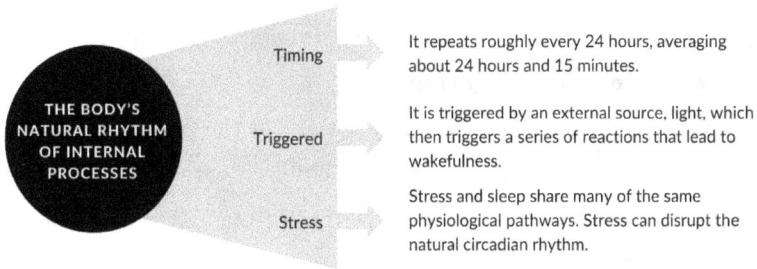

THE BODY'S NATURAL RHYTHM OF INTERNAL PROCESSES

Timing → It repeats roughly every 24 hours, averaging about 24 hours and 15 minutes.

Triggered → It is triggered by an external source, light, which then triggers a series of reactions that lead to wakefulness.

Stress → Stress and sleep share many of the same physiological pathways. Stress can disrupt the natural circadian rhythm.

The CLOCK and CRY1 genes are central to maintaining these rhythms. Whether we have these genes in variant form or the normal form, they can be impacted by stress or inflammation, and the circadian rhythm can be disrupted. For example, children with ADHD often experience delayed melatonin production, the hormone that signals the body to prepare for sleep. This delay can make it challenging for them to fall asleep at a typical bedtime and may lead to additional issues such as fragmented sleep or waking earlier than desired.

There are three common sleep challenges, and children with ADHD can exhibit one, two, or all three of these types of insomnia:

1. Sleep Onset Challenges

These challenges are often tied to increased anxiety levels and overactive minds—both influenced by serotonin production and its conversion to melatonin. Serotonin serves as a precursor to melatonin, the hormone that signals the brain to prepare for sleep. Genetic variations in enzymes like tryptophan hydroxylase (TPH2, as covered in Step Five – Calm) or melatonin receptor genes can disrupt or delay this conversion, complicating the sleep process.

Pre-bedtime activities also play a significant role. Evaluating your child's routines during the hour before bed can provide valuable insights. While it's widely recognized that screen time before bed can be particularly disruptive for children with ADHD, exceptions exist (see our discussion on this later in the Step). We also understand that limiting screens at the end of a long day might not feel achievable for every family.

However, since many ADHD brains already struggle with circadian rhythm regulation, the blue light emitted by screens can further exacerbate these issues. Therefore, consider whether action-packed TV shows or stimulating video games are beneficial in preparing your child for restful sleep.

2. Sleep Maintenance Challenges

These issues may be related to disruptions in the body's ability to regulate arousal and relaxation, often seen in children with ADHD. The body's arousal-relaxation balance is regulated by the autonomic nervous system, with the sympathetic nervous system (SNS) managing arousal (fight-or-flight) and the parasympathetic nervous system (PNS) promoting relaxation (rest-and-digest). In ADHD, there may be heightened SNS activity or difficulty activating the PNS, leading to an inability to stay in a restful state through the night.

Parents may need to act as detectives to explore potential triggers. For example, is your child waking up due to external stimuli (e.g., noises, light) or internal factors (e.g., nightmares, blood sugar dips, or stress-related hormonal fluctuations)? Tools like a sleep diary or observing patterns in their diet or bedtime routine can offer valuable insights.

3. Early Waking

Waking 30 minutes or more before the desired wake time can stem from an inability to maintain sleep. This may be influenced by genetic factors beyond sleep-related genes, such as those involved in serotonin metabolism or cortisol regulation. For instance, increased cortisol levels in the early morning can prematurely rouse a child from sleep.

To assess whether early waking is problematic, you can evaluate your child's sleep quality and quantity by their morning behaviors. Do they wake up well-rested and ready to start the day, or do they want to head back to bed or collapse on the couch? If the latter, their sleep quantity and quality are likely insufficient.

Overall, sleep quality can be a challenge, and even with "enough" sleep, ADHD brains can have trouble feeling rested. A sleep chart is a great way to assess these common sleep challenges with your child.

Three Common Sleep Challenges and ADHD

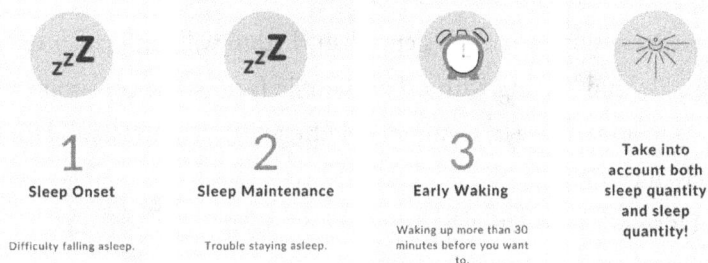

1	**2**	**3**	Take into account both sleep quantity and sleep quantity!
Sleep Onset	Sleep Maintenance	Early Waking	
Difficulty falling asleep.	Trouble staying asleep.	Waking up more than 30 minutes before you want to.	

Resetting Circadian Rhythm

Establishing good sleep hygiene practices is crucial in mitigating sleep issues; those practices don't just start at bedtime. One of the most effective strategies is morning sunlight exposure.

Natural light helps reset the circadian rhythm by signaling to the brain that it's time to wake. Early morning light exposure helps suppress melatonin production and encourages cortisol release, preparing the body and mind for the day ahead. To help regulate your child's internal clock, aim for 10–30 minutes of outdoor activity in the morning. Eat breakfast on your deck or in your backyard, or start the day with a quick walk together.

If you live at a latitude where early morning light comes after your child is already on the way to school, consider using a seasonal affective disorder (SAD) light. These lights mimic natural sunlight and provide wavelengths like blue, green, and purple, which are particularly effective for regulating circadian rhythms. Position the SAD light at eye level, about 12–24 inches away, and use it for 20–30 minutes while your child eats breakfast or gets ready for school. Avoid looking directly into the light, as indirect exposure is sufficient for its benefits. This can be especially helpful during darker winter months when natural light is limited.

Reducing exposure to artificial light, particularly blue light from screens, is essential in the evenings, especially for ADHD brains. Blue light's morning benefit of interfering with melatonin production is not beneficial in the evening when it makes it harder to fall asleep. Consider implementing a "no screens" rule at least an hour before bedtime—note exceptions to follow—and using warm, dim lighting in the evening.

Note that resetting your child's circadian rhythm will not impact only their sleep. This rhythm—along with other lifestyle factors like consistent feeding times—has an impact on a large number of physiological processes and functions in the body, including:

- Hormone production and release

- Metabolism and digestion

- Immune system function

- Body temperature regulation

- DNA and cellular repair

- Detoxification and inflammation

- Cardiovascular function

- Mood and cognitive function

So, while your primary goal in resetting your child's circadian rhythm may be to promote sounder, higher-quality, and more consistent sleep, know that you are doing your child's body well in many crucial areas!

Resetting Circadian Rhythm

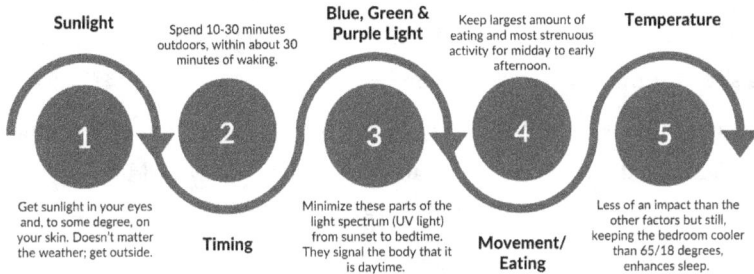

Sunlight	Spend 10-30 minutes outdoors, within about 30 minutes of waking.	**Blue, Green & Purple Light**	Keep largest amount of eating and most strenuous activity for midday to early afternoon.	**Temperature**
1	**2**	**3**	**4**	**5**
Get sunlight in your eyes and, to some degree, on your skin. Doesn't matter the weather; get outside.	**Timing**	Minimize these parts of the light spectrum (UV light) from sunset to bedtime. They signal the body that it is daytime.	**Movement/ Eating**	Less of an impact than the other factors but still, keeping the bedroom cooler than 65/18 degrees, enhances sleep.

Sleep Environment

Creating a conducive sleep environment can also significantly affect sleep quality. The bedroom should be dark—if possible, avoid night lights—and a cool and quiet sanctuary for sleep. Use blackout curtains to help block out external light and a white noise machine to mask background noise. Set the room temperature to around 65°F (18°C), which can help facilitate the body's natural drop in temperature that promotes sleep.

Additionally, establishing a consistent bedtime routine can signal your child's body that it's time to wind down. To start with, try to keep waking and bedtimes consistent. Even on the weekends, if you can avoid deviating from those times by more than an hour, you will likely find it helpful for your child's sleep routine.

An exception might be during the teen years. Due to biological and developmental changes in their bodies, teens need more sleep than adults or younger children. If they are in the conventional school system, they must get up early to get to class on time. That means they may need some catch-up sleep time on the weekends. However, have them avoid getting to bed too late and only extend the morning sleep-in by a couple of hours at most.

Activities like reading a book, following a calming meditative practice, tapping (more on tapping in Step Five – Calm), or taking a warm bath can help ease the transition to sleep.

Various tools and techniques can further improve sleep quality and quantity. Relaxation exercises, such as deep breathing or progressive muscle relaxation, can help calm the mind and body before bed. Guided imagery or bedtime stories can also provide a soothing transition to sleep. Remember to model the behaviors you want to see in your child. Quiet yourself in the evening, stay off your devices, and have a sleep routine that works for you.

When my (Alicia) kids were younger, at bedtime, we would settle them, turn off the lights, and I would begin creating a story, with my children as the main characters. The stories always included aspects of how each child's day had gone. Not only was the time fun and calming, but it also opened the door for some excellent dialogue before the kids went to sleep.

Another bedtime technique I used was progressive relaxation, in which we alternated contracting and relaxing different parts of our bodies. We'd start by relaxing our toes and work our way up the body to our faces. Sometimes, I still do this before I go to sleep, and I still find it fun and relaxing.

As mentioned in the guidelines for resetting circadian rhythm, monitoring technology use before bedtime is essential. Encourage non-screen activities like drawing, playing with non-electronic toys, or listening to calming music.

Dr. Kendall-Reed also highly recommends listening to binaural beats (and, after personal use, we concur!). Binaural beats are not music, per se, but are an experience of listening to two different sound frequencies simultaneously. This auditory phenomenon comes in various combinations (e.g., frequencies that help with calming or focus), and when sustained for a length of time, they can alter your brain wave activity. You can easily find relaxing, meditative, or anxiety-reducing binaural beats music on YouTube or Spotify. Ensure you listen to it with earphones or headphones so each side of your brain listens to the specific beat.

Many techniques can be used with your child to support them when going to sleep. We encourage you and them to use your imaginations, as creating a bedtime routine that your child looks forward to can significantly impact their willingness to go to bed and their sleep quality once they are there!

Why Screen Time Before Bed Might Be Helpful for Some Children with ADHD

It might seem counterintuitive, but there are several reasons why some children with ADHD might find it easier to fall asleep after playing video games or watching TV, even though these activities are generally discouraged before bedtime. Here are a few key factors that could explain this scenario:

1. Hyperfocus as a Calming Mechanism

- Children with ADHD often experience racing thoughts or difficulty winding down at the end of the day. Video games or TV shows can help them hyperfocus, temporarily quieting the brain's "noise" and providing a singular focus point. This can mimic a calming effect, making it easier for the child to relax.

2. Dopamine Regulation

- As we've mentioned, ADHD is often associated with low levels of dopamine, a neurotransmitter involved in motivation, attention, and reward. Video games and engaging TV content can trigger a temporary dopamine release, providing a momentary sense of pleasure or satisfaction. For some children, this boost might regulate their brain's reward system just enough to help them transition into a more relaxed state conducive to sleep.

- However, dopamine's effects are highly individual and context-dependent. While increasing dopamine can help in certain circumstances—such as improving focus or reducing impulsivity—excessive dopamine, particularly close to bedtime, can disrupt the brain's ability to wind down and interfere with sleep onset. This highlights the delicate balance required: More or less dopamine can be beneficial depending on the situation, but finding the "just right" amount for your child is key.

- Encourage mindful use of activities that trigger dopamine release, ensuring they support healthy routines without creating dependencies or inadvertently making it harder for your child to relax at day's end.

3. Stimulation-Induced Regulation

- Paradoxically, some children with ADHD need a certain level of stimulation to feel calm. Known as the "stimulation paradox," the engaging nature of video games or TV might help regulate their underactive brain. By engaging their attention, these activities can prevent the child from becoming restless or overwhelmed by their thoughts before bedtime.

4. Sensory Overload Reduction

- For children who struggle with sensory sensitivities or an overstimulated nervous system, the consistent and predictable sensory input from a TV show or video game can feel comforting. The repetitive sound, visuals, and storyline create a structured environment that may help them wind down.

5. Association and Routine

- If a child has developed a habit of watching TV or playing video games before bed, it may have become a conditioned part of their bedtime routine. Their brain might associate these activities with winding down, regardless of the content.

Caveats and Concerns

Though it may seem some children benefit from pre-bed screen exposure, we have several concerns.

Blue Light Disruption

- The blue light emitted by screens suppresses melatonin production, which signals the body it's time to sleep. While video games or TV might help a child relax initially, the suppression of melatonin can delay the natural sleep cycle and lead to poorer sleep quality in the long term.

Overstimulation Risk

- While some children feel calmer after gaming or watching TV, others may become overstimulated. Fast-paced content, bright lights, and immersive gameplay can make it harder for their brains to switch gears and settle down.

Dependency and Sleep Crutches

- Relying on TV or gaming as a sleep aid can create a dependency. Over time, this could prevent the child from learning other, more sustainable calming techniques, such as mindfulness, reading, or calming music.

Alternative Strategies

For parents whose children rely on TV or video games to fall asleep, consider offering other tools that might achieve similar effects without the drawbacks:

- **White Noise or Calming Sounds:** Apps or machines with consistent background noise can mimic the predictable TV input without the blue light.

- **Audiobooks or Guided Meditations:** These offer a single point of focus, like TV, but are less stimulating.

- **Transitional Time:** Gradually wean the child off screens before bed by setting a specific time limit and then transitioning to less stimulating activities.

Understanding your child's individual needs and responses is critical. If video games or TV genuinely help your child fall asleep, monitor their overall sleep quality and try to balance this habit with healthier long-term strategies.

Supplements to Support Sound Sleep

Once sleep hygiene and other lifestyle shifts have been tried, supplements can be considered if sleep is still not optimal. Provided a potential supplement is not contraindicated with any medications your child may take (check with your doctor or pharmacist to be sure), supplements can be used to improve sleep for children with ADHD.

Melatonin is a popular supplement that can help regulate sleep-wake cycles, particularly for those with delayed sleep phase disorder. We like the time-release or slow-release versions. Talk with a healthcare provider to determine the appropriate dosage and timing.

Lactium®, a milk protein hydrolysate, can help reduce stress and anxiety by calming the nervous system, leading to better sleep. L-theanine, an amino acid in green tea, can enhance relaxation and improve sleep quality. Gamma-aminobu-tyric acid (GABA) is a neurotransmitter that helps reduce neuronal excitability, promoting a sense of calm and aiding sleep. Child-safe, traditionally used herbal supplements like passion flower, chamomile, lemon balm, and valerian root can also be beneficial.

With any sleep-supporting supplements, watch for daytime tiredness or irri-tability and adjust or discontinue supplement use if necessary.

TRAVELER ASSISTANCE

We usually recommend that caffeine—found in coffee, tea, chocolate, and some energy drinks—be avoided with children to protect sleep, yet some parents find it helpful for ADHD. Here's a brief look at why it might work, the caveats, and practical tips:

Why Caffeine Might Work for ADHD

- **Stimulant Effect**: Like ADHD medications, caffeine increases dopamine and norepinephrine availability, improving focus and im-pulse control.

- **Normalizing Arousal Levels**: ADHD brains often seek stimulation. Small doses of caffeine may help meet this need, improving attention and calming hyperactivity.

- **Alternative to Medication**: For families hesitant to use stimulants, low doses of caffeine (e.g., a small amount of tea or coffee) may provide mild benefits.

Caveats and Concerns

- **Overstimulation**: Too much caffeine can cause jitters, anxiety, and worsen sleep—already a challenge for many children with ADHD.

- **Detoxification Challenges:** Caffeine can slow down Phase 1 detoxifi-cation, potentially exacerbating issues for individuals with a genetically slower Phase 1 (More on this in Step Four – Detox). This may lead to difficulty processing toxins and increased sensitivity to caffeine's effects.

- **Short-Term Effects**: Caffeine only lasts a few hours and may lead to a "crash," reducing focus later.

- **Tolerance and Dependence**: Regular use may require higher doses and lead to withdrawal symptoms if stopped.

- **Sugary Additives**: Avoid sodas and energy drinks high in sugar, which can negate caffeine's benefits.

Practical Tips

- **Start Small**: Begin with a half-cup of coffee or a small piece of dark chocolate and observe the effects.

- **Timing Matters**: Offer caffeine in the morning or early afternoon to avoid sleep disruption.

- **Choose Whole Sources**: Opt for natural options like green tea, which contains calming L-theanine.

- **Consult Your Provider**: Discuss caffeine use with your child's doctor, especially if combined with ADHD medications.

- **Track**: If you test caffeine with your child, keep track of any Sleep/Mood connections. I (Alicia), for example, am highly sensitive to caffeine. If I have caffeine in the morning, I might be awake for the next two nights.

Final Thoughts:

While caffeine can mimic some of the effects of ADHD medications and may be helpful for certain children, it's not a one-size-fits-all solution. The variability in how children respond to caffeine—at least, in part, a function of their neurotransmitter and detoxification genes—underscores the importance of individualized approaches to ADHD management. For most children, a holistic strategy that includes diet, sleep, physical activity, and behavioral interventions will offer more sustainable benefits than caffeine.

REST STOP

Take 10 minutes of calm to reflect on these questions:

Your Child's Sleep Environment: Consider the sensory aspects of your child's sleep space (light, noise, comfort). Are there adjustments you can make to create a more restful environment?

Sleep Struggles and Solutions: Are there recurring issues like bedtime anxiety or difficulty winding down? Reflect on how you respond to these struggles—are current strategies effective, or could new approaches help ease the transition to sleep?

Next, take 10 minutes of quiet, either sitting or slowly walking. Clear your mind and listen. Jot down or tell Siri to "make a note" of any thoughts that arise. These insights may provide clues to the reasons behind your answers and reveal potential problematic thinking that can guide you forward. Those clues, in turn, will reveal potential problematic thinking and can provide great direction on moving forward with the recommendations in this Step that would be the easiest to implement or fit best for your family!

ROADWORK

Create Your Child's Sleep Sanctuary

Materials:

- Notebook or digital device

- Pen

- Timer or alarm to help with scheduling routines

Directions:

1. **Morning Light Routine**: Schedule 10-30 minutes of outdoor activity in the morning to reset your circadian rhythm. Note the time and activity in your notebook.

2. **Evening Light Management**: For most children, enforce a "no screens" rule at least one hour before bed. Use warm, dim lighting.

3. **Bedroom Environment**: Ensure the room is dark, cool, and quiet.

Consider blackout curtains or white noise. Note any changes.

4. **Bedtime Routine**: Establish a consistent routine with calming activities like reading or a warm bath. Write it down.

5. **Supplementation**: Consult a healthcare provider about supplements for sleep support. Note any recommendations.

Creating a personalized sleep plan helps you systematically improve your child's sleep quality and track what works.

SOUVENIR

After evaluating your family's sleep routines, choose a Step Three – Sleep souvenir that fits:

- Sleep mask

- Warm flannelette pillowcases

- Room-darkening shades

- White noise machine

- Binaural beats before bed

- Total bedroom makeover

- A new bedtime storybook

Find what works best for your family and start improving your sleep immediately.

Next, we'll explore detoxification, a vital body process, and its crucial role in managing ADHD.

Chapter 7

Core Step Four - Detox

"The natural healing force within each of us is the greatest force in getting well."

- Hippocrates

SUMMARY - Travel Size Version

I (Brenda) am thinking back ... way back. I'm preparing dinner when our children burst in from the vacant lot behind our townhouse complex, their hands covered in dirt and our missing gardening and household maintenance tools in tow, all while wearing big smiles. I'm happy they've had fun outside and relieved that no one has pounded a thumbnail with the hammer or twisted an ankle on a root. However, I can't shake the worry about the invisible toxins they might have been exposed to.

Environmental toxins are everywhere—in air, soil, water, and food— from the chemicals the township sprayed to keep mosquitoes and blackberry bushes at bay to the fumes from the dry cleaners up the street. These toxins can significantly impact anyone, especially children with ADHD. Understanding how to minimize these exposures and support your child's natural detoxification processes can make a world of difference.

Detoxification Genes

As usual, we'll start with some science. We'll examine two genes that assist in Phase 1 detoxification and three that are involved in Phase 2 detoxification. Think of this section as a quick guide to reducing your child's exposure to harmful substances and enhancing their body's natural ability to detoxify.

By Detoxification, You Mean What???

Next, we will clarify what detoxification means. Imagine your child's body as a house that needs regular cleaning. Detoxification is the process of sweeping out dust and taking out the trash. Some children, however, are like houses with tricky nooks and crannies where dirt tends to get stuck, making regular cleaning a bit more challenging. Genetic factors can hinder their bodies' detoxification ability, so we need to provide them with extra support.

Creating a Toxin-Free Environment

Creating a toxin-free environment may seem daunting, but it becomes manageable when broken down into steps. We'll discuss ways to support detoxification by minimizing exposure to common toxins found in everyday items and give tips on helping your child's body improve detoxification in general.

INFORMATION CENTER

The Impact of Detoxification on ADHD and Gene Expression

The science of detoxification is fascinating and crucial, especially for children with ADHD. Detoxification is your body's natural way of eliminating harmful substances, but genetic changes, lifestyle, and diet can affect how well this process works.

The Centers for Disease Control and Prevention (CDC) has identified an average of 212 chemicals in people's blood or urine, and the Environmental Protection Agency (EPA) states that an ordinary person (e.g., someone not exposed to chemicals in their work) can encounter up to 84,000 manufactured chemicals daily.

Before diving into detox genes, let's discuss the liver, a powerhouse organ responsible for metabolizing drugs and pollutants. The liver can regenerate, store vitamins, and regulate blood sugar levels. It is crucial to support it with a healthy diet, physical activity, and hydration. When the liver doesn't filter toxins properly, they can accumulate in the body, potentially leading to neuroinflammation or brain function disruptions, which can affect attention, impulse control, and executive function in children with ADHD.

Though more research is needed, supporting detoxification through diet, hydration, and reducing toxin exposure may alleviate ADHD symptoms for some individuals. This Step explores the epigenetics of liver detoxification pathways, offering insights into how your child's liver processes toxins and why a well-functioning detox system may help manage ADHD symptoms.

First, let's examine the genetic markers supporting liver detox. The **CYP1A2** gene, part of the cytochrome P450 family, governs the metabolism of chemicals, food, drugs, and toxins. Variations in this gene affect how quickly your child processes substances, impacting their sensitivity to environmental toxins. Another critical gene is **CYP3A4**, which is also involved in metabolizing a wide range of substances. Variations in this gene influence detox efficiency.

Although over 50 members of this family of enzymes exist, 90% of drugs are metabolized by CYP1A2 and CYP3A4, making them the most prominent. These two genes also play a crucial role in the metabolism of xenobiotics (e.g., carcinogens, drugs, environmental pollutants, food additives, hydrocarbons, and pesticides).

Phase 1 of detoxification plays an initial role in the breakdown of these compounds, primarily soluble in fat and predominantly stored inside our fat cells. These compounds contribute to a wide range of symptoms, from inflammation to toxicity.

What does this mean for your child with ADHD? If your child doesn't have a lot of adipocytes (fat cells) in which the toxins can be stored, those toxins may accumulate in other body parts containing fat. As the brain is composed of approximately 60% fat, when a child has an abundance of toxins and poor processing of those toxins, it is possible to see some connection between poor detoxification and a challenging impact on brain functioning.

In the second detoxification phase, we encounter three additional genes: **SOD2**, **GSTP1**, and **NQO1**. These genes are involved in converting those toxic substrates into a water-soluble form that can be more easily eliminated from the body.

SOD2 encodes an enzyme called superoxide dismutase, which protects cells from oxidative damage. Changes in this gene can affect the body's ability to neutralize harmful free radicals, potentially exacerbating oxidative stress and ADHD symptoms. Imagine that the paint on your car has been oxidized. It is no longer shiny; you can even see parts of the vehicle where the paint is completely dissolved and the metal is rusted. This rusting process is equivalent to what can happen in our cells when oxidation occurs.

The GSTP1 gene encodes for glutathione S-transferase, an enzyme involved in detoxifying harmful compounds by conjugating them with glutathione. Variations in this gene can impact the body's ability to detoxify environmental toxins, leading to an accumulation of harmful substances.

Lastly, the NQO1 gene encodes for NAD(P)H quinone dehydrogenase, an enzyme that protects cells from oxidative stress by detoxifying quinones. Variations in this gene can affect the efficiency of this detoxification pathway, potentially increasing the risk of toxin-related health issues.

SNP Peek - Detoxification Genes

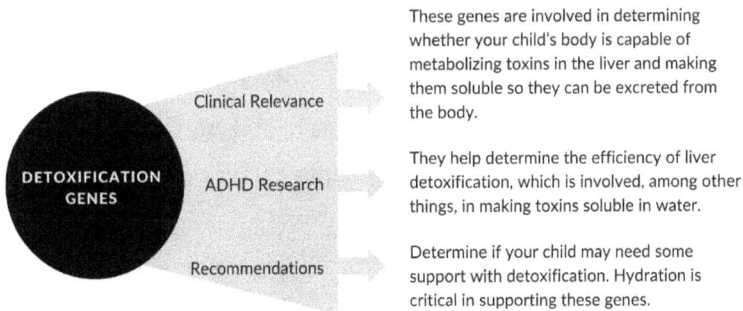

DETOXIFICATION GENES

Clinical Relevance

These genes are involved in determining whether your child's body is capable of metabolizing toxins in the liver and making them soluble so they can be excreted from the body.

ADHD Research

They help determine the efficiency of liver detoxification, which is involved, among other things, in making toxins soluble in water.

Recommendations

Determine if your child may need some support with detoxification. Hydration is critical in supporting these genes.

If your child's body odor is noticeably strong or unpleasant, it could be a sign of potential health issues. Though the skin is indeed an elimination organ, the odor could indicate that toxins are being released through the skin due to inadequate elimination through other pathways. Effective detoxification relies on regular bowel movements and urination, so if constipation or infrequent urination is present, it may suggest that the body's detox systems aren't working as efficiently. To support detoxification, ensure your child urinates and has bowel movements daily.

Keeping "Detoxification" Simple

We understand that the detoxification process can be pretty challenging to understand, so we'll help you make a link between these detoxification pathways and ADHD.

Some studies suggest children with ADHD may have trouble detoxifying certain environmental toxins, such as heavy metals (e.g., lead, mercury, cadmium), pesticides, and other chemicals, which can affect brain function. Genetic variations in detoxification enzymes may lead to slower detoxification, allowing neurotoxic substances to accumulate.

Understanding these genetic factors helps us appreciate why some children may be more sensitive to environmental toxins and how we can support their detoxification processes.

Environmental Toxins

Heavy metals, pesticides, and food additives are common environmental toxins that can impact children with ADHD. Lead exposure, for instance, has been linked to increased ADHD risk. These toxins come from everyday sources like old paint, plumbing pipes, contaminated soil, non-organic produce, processed foods, and poor indoor air quality.

Creating a toxin-free environment at home is ideal, but a more realistic goal is a toxin-minimized environment. Start by improving air quality—open windows, add air-purifying plants, and consider air purifiers.

Avoid Teflon cookware. When heated to high temperatures, it can release toxic fumes containing perfluorooctanoic acid (PFOA) and other chemicals, contributing to indoor air pollution and posing health risks. Instead, use ceramic, cast iron, or stainless steel. Minimize your use of plastic containers, especially in the microwave.

Other ways to foster a toxin-minimized environment that will hopefully avoid the worsening of ADHD symptoms?

- Replace conventional candles, plug-ins, and air fresheners with home-made sprays, beeswax or soy candles, and diffusers that use high-quality essential oils—provided you don't have susceptible pets, as many essential oils are not pet-safe—or simply go scent-free.

- Ditch dryer sheets in favor of wool dryer balls scented with essential oils.

- Swap out PVC shower curtains for fabric or PVC-free alternatives to avoid chemical off-gassing.

- Choose non-toxic cleaning supplies from brands such as Seventh Generation and Norwex.

- Consider buying used furniture and household items made from natural fibers like wood and wool instead of plastic.

- Clean regularly, remove shoes indoors, and use doormats to reduce allergens and dust.

- Switch to beauty and skincare products that don't contribute to indoor air pollution.

- To avoid pesticide residues on non-organic produce and in household pest control products, choose organic or locally grown, non-sprayed produce as often as possible. Also, deal with household pests and outdoor weeds as naturally as possible.

- Avoid food additives, such as artificial colors and preservatives, as they have been shown to worsen hyperactivity and inattention in susceptible children.

For more guidance, the Environmental Working Group (EWG) offers resources like the Dirty Dozen list for produce, which identifies fruits and vegetables with the highest pesticide residues, and the Skin Deep database for checking the safety of personal care products. These resources can help you make informed choices to reduce your child's exposure to harmful toxins.

Remember, these are guidelines. Don't try to implement them all at once. The bottom line is to take it one step at a time and prioritize changes that resonate most with your family.

I (Alicia) remember telling my husband that our microwave was too old and not worth testing for safety (e.g., potential radiation leakage, degraded components). He got rid of it. When the kids came into the kitchen looking to "nuke" a quick snack, I told them to use the stove. It was a "fun" moment in our household ... but they did get used to the change!

Enhancing the Detoxification Process

Supporting your child's detoxification processes doesn't stop at creating a toxin-reduced environment. Several additional practices and techniques can help enhance detoxification.

- **Dry brushing** stimulates the lymphatic system, promoting the removal of toxins through the skin. Before a bath or shower, use a natural bristle brush to gently brush your child's skin in long, upward strokes toward the heart. For specific directions, see this Step's Traveler Assistance.

- **Saunas**, whether traditional or infrared, can help eliminate toxins through sweat. If you choose to use a sauna, ensure your child stays hydrated and consult a healthcare provider before using it, especially for younger children.

- **Castor oil packs** are another effective detoxification technique. Apply a generous amount of castor oil to a stack of 4-6 8-inch square pieces of flannel or cotton cloth (the "pack"), place the pack on your child's abdomen (ensuring you're covering the liver/gallbladder area on the upper right quadrant of the abdomen), cover it with plastic wrap, and apply a heating pad for about 30 minutes. Initially, repeat the process for six weeks, 4-6 consecutive days/week. This method can support liver function and improve digestion. If your child is older and menstruating, do not use heat during their period, as it can increase flow. Find more details on castor oil pack use in the Traveler's Assistance section of Core Step Six - Inflammation.

- Relaxing **Epsom salt baths** are another way to enhance detoxification. Add a cup or two of Epsom salt to a warm bath and let your child soak for 20-30 minutes. The magnesium in Epsom salts can help reduce stress, relax muscles, and support detoxification.

- **Movement** is also a key component of detoxification. Physical activity helps speed the flow of lymph fluid, which carries nutrients to cells and removes waste material. Encourage your child to exercise regularly, whether playing outside, riding their bike, or participating in sports. The goal is to keep their body moving and their lymphatic system active.

- Don't forget about **sleep**. Detoxification occurs while we sleep. Did you know our normal flora produces about 2 liters of gas daily? And all of it needs to come out? Well, if you are like me (Alicia), a person that grew up not allowed to fart in public, guess what? All of that gas will come out while you sleep. Making passing gas a regularly accepted part of the family lifestyle is better!

- **Relaxation and deep breathing** can support detoxification while also supporting sleep.

- **Nutrition and hydration** also play a significant role in detoxification. Ensure your child gets enough water and fiber-rich foods to support the body's natural ability to detox through the skin, lungs, kidneys, and bowels.

- Remember to support **regular bowel movements**! The daily elimination of poop is an essential detoxification method. Work with your child so they don't get constipated, and have 1-3 BMs daily!

Will these changes make a difference? Yes, absolutely, for most children and adults, particularly those with challenging detoxification genes!

Supplements to Support Detoxification

Supplements like glutathione, N-acetylcysteine (NAC), and DIM (diindolyl-methane) can further support liver detox.

Glutathione is an excellent antioxidant that helps neutralize free radicals and supports the liver's detoxification processes. N-acetylcysteine (NAC) is a precursor to glutathione and can enhance its production in the body.

Please note that though both these supplements support phase 2 detoxification, NAC crosses the blood-brain barrier, while glutathione does not. Although they have different mechanisms of functioning in the body, they both support detoxification and inflammation. We typically recommend that glutathione and NAC be taken together on an empty stomach. If your child's stomach gets upset with these supplements, they can take them with a small rice cracker or a bit of fruit, but no protein.

DIM (diindolylmethane), a compound found in cruciferous vegetables like broccoli and Brussels sprouts, supports phase 1 of liver detoxification. While cruciferous vegetables are generally highly recommended for their health benefits, including their ability to aid detoxification, certain individuals may need to be cautious about consuming them in their raw form. If your phase 1 detoxification is already overly fast relative to phase 2 (as influenced by your SNPs), raw cruciferous vegetables could further accelerate phase 1, potentially creating an imbalance and leading to the buildup of intermediate toxins. In such cases, working with a healthcare provider to balance detox pathways is key, and cooked cruciferous vegetables or alternative methods of obtaining DIM may be better suited for you.

Choose high-quality supplements (i.e., Good Manufacturing Practices, a DIN number) and consult your healthcare provider to determine if the supplement is appropriate and what dosage and regimen are correct for your child.

For our last case study in this Step, meet Hana, a bright and fun 8-year-old who came to us because she had vitiligo, a condition in which immune cells destroy the cells that make melanin or brown pigment. The skin begins to turn white, often with white patches appearing across different parts of the body. As part of our intake process, Hana's parents also told us that Hana had ADHD.

After addressing her detox pathways and optimizing diet, sleep, and movement, Hana's vitiligo and ADHD symptoms improved. Her focus in school increased, and even her teacher noticed the changes. After pausing supplements for a week, Hana's symptoms worsened, confirming the benefits of continuing her personalized regimen. Today, her mom says, "We will never stop what we are doing. It truly works for Hana."

TRAVELER ASSISTANCE

Dry brushing is a technique that involves gently brushing the skin with a dry, soft-bristled brush to promote circulation and exfoliation. Because of its effect on the lymphatic system, it can also enhance immune support. Here's a step-by-step guide:

1. Prepare:

- Consult a pediatrician before dry brushing, especially if your child has skin conditions or sensitivities.

- Select a brush with a comfortable handle and soft, natural bristles suitable for delicate skin. Ensure the brush is clean and dry before each use.

- Find a comfortable, warm space where your child feels relaxed. Explain the process to them to ensure they are comfortable and willing.

2. Brushing:

- Begin at the soles of the feet, using gentle, upward strokes toward the heart. Repeat 5–10 times on each leg. Do this on the inner leg and inner arms, where the skin is thinner.

- Brush from the hands up the arms toward the shoulders, always moving in the direction of the heart. Use light pressure and repeat 5–10 times on each arm.

- For the back, brush from the lower back upward toward the shoulders. On the torso, use gentle strokes from the abdomen upward toward the chest.

- Avoid brushing over sensitive areas, such as the face, neck, or any areas with cuts, rashes, or irritations.

- Keep sessions short, around 2–3 minutes, and observe your child's response. If your child enjoys it, dry brushing can be done 1–2 times weekly.

3. Post-Brushing Care:
- After brushing, you can bathe your child to remove exfoliated skin cells. Then, apply a gentle moisturizer to keep the skin hydrated.

- Always monitor your child's skin for any signs of irritation. If redness or discomfort occurs, discontinue use.

This gentle approach to dry brushing can be a soothing addition to your child's routine. It supports the immune system, promotes detoxification, relaxation, and healthy skin, and is a comforting practice that can enhance your child's overall wellness.

REST STOP

It's time for parents to take a break and digest information! Take 10 minutes of calm to Rest with the following questions:

1. **Toxins in the Home Environment:** What everyday products or habits in your home might contribute to a less-than-ideal detox environment (e.g., ultra-processed foods, cleaning supplies, deep-dyed bedding, plastics)? What small, manageable steps could you take to create a cleaner, more supportive environment for natural detoxification?

2. **Your Child's Detox Pathways**: How does your child typically respond to changes in diet, routine, or physical environment? Are there signs that their body might struggle to detoxify efficiently (e.g., frequent headaches, digestive issues, skin problems)? Reflect on whether adjusting their diet, physical activity, bowel movements, urination, or sleep could provide support.

3. **Your Child's Hydration**: How much water does your child consume daily? Is it enough to support their body's removal of toxins? Does your child consume drinks other than water? You might want to check if these beverages support their detoxification pathways.

Next, Stop for 10 minutes of quiet (sitting or slowly walking). Keep your mind as clear and open as possible, and just listen. Jot down or tell Siri to "make a note" of any responses that may arise. Because you've taken time to ponder calmly and quietly, these responses will most likely be less off-the-cuff and from a deeper level. They can give you clues as to the reasons behind your answers! Those clues, in turn, will reveal potential problematic thinking and can provide great direction on moving forward with the recommendations in this Step that would be the easiest to implement or fit best for your family!

ROADWORK
Create Your Child's Detox Action Plan
Materials:
- Notebook or digital device, pen

Directions:

1. **Identify Toxins:** List common sources of toxins in your home (e.g., cleaning supplies, food additives, air fresheners).

2. **Plan for Replacement:** Note safer alternatives (e.g., non-toxic cleaning brands, organic produce, essential oil diffusers).

3. **Implement Detox Techniques:** Schedule regular dry brushing, castor oil pack use, sauna sessions, or Epsom salt baths.

4. **Encourage Movement:** Plan daily physical activities to promote lymphatic flow.

5. **Supplements:** Consult a healthcare provider about appropriate detox supplements for your child.

This action plan helps you systematically reduce toxin exposure and support your child's natural detoxification processes, making it easier to manage ADHD symptoms.

SOUVENIR

For this Step's Souvenir, we encourage you to give yourself and your child the gift of improved detoxification!

Enhancing toxin removal involves supporting our "emunctory" organs—lungs, bowels, kidneys, and skin—which our body uses for elimination and excretion. In other words, we encourage you to talk with your child about pooping, peeing, sweating, and deep breathing.

How many times a day does your child poop? What does it look like? Is it like a nice light brown color sausage that comes out smoothly? Does your child strain? And be open to this conversation. It's worth it!

Next, look at how much water your child drinks and how many times/how much they pee each day. What color is the urine? Is it a bit yellowish in the morning, and is it lighter in color as the day progresses?

What about sweat? Many toxins come out through the skin. I (Alicia) remember a mom of an adolescent with ADHD who said that her teen smelled "like a goat." She said it was rather disgusting. Discuss with your child how toxins come out through sweat as well.

Finally, breathing is another way of removing toxins. After all, we inhale oxygen and exhale carbon dioxide. When we consciously do some deep breathing, we don't only relax; we also get rid of toxins as we exhale and refill our lungs with fresh air as we inhale.

Keep a journal of all these ways of getting rid of toxins, and review changes with your child as their detoxification system is better supported.

Next, we'll explore Calm and how it impacts ADHD. We'll look at strategies to manage Calm and support overall health.

Chapter 8

Core Step Five - Calm

"The greatest weapon against stress is our ability to choose one thought over another."

- William James, author of The Principles of Psychology

S UMMARY - Travel Size Version

It's the last Saturday before school starts, and you're in the middle of a big-box store. Your child is having a tantrum over which pencil case to choose. The noise, the lights, the length of time since their last snack, and the sheer number of pencil case choices have overwhelmed them. Fists are flailing. The previously nicely organized display is now mainly on the floor, and your child is yelling at the top of their lungs that they "hate you!" In short, stress has played a role in moving dopamine from the prefrontal cortex to the anterior striatum, and they have gone from being able to focus to being "all over the map."

You feel the familiar twinge of anxiety in the pit of your gut and a little tightening in your throat, and, along with fighting embarrassment at the scene unfolding in front of you, you wonder, "Is there ever going to be a way to help my child find calm amid the chaos?" We've already covered an array of suggestions in the book that will impact events like this. Still, the power of mindfulness and meditation—tools we'll cover in this Step—is significant in how they can help transform the foundation of calmness from which your child experiences the world.

Stress Management Genes

We'll continue with the critical and enlightening world of epigenetics and start this Step with how genes influence our ability to find calm. We'll look at a couple of genes that regulate dopamine production and then cover two genes related to serotonin production. Next, we'll cover a gene that plays a significant role in cortisol regulation along the Hypothalamic-Pituitary-Adrenal (HPA) axis and finally give you information on a bonus gene related to GABA production.

Mindfulness

Imagine mindfulness as a way to help your child hit the pause button on their racing thoughts. It's about teaching them to focus on the present moment, whether they're feeling hyperactive or weighed down by intrusive thoughts. We'll present simple practices like deep breathing that can work wonders in helping your child calm their mind and get in touch with their body.

Routines

Routines are another key element to helping your child have fewer situational mismatches with how their neurodiverse brain functions. Think of routines as the scaffolding that supports your child's day. Flexibility within routines, however, is vital. We'll lay out several ways to strike a balance between consistency and adaptability.

Emotional Regulation

While this whole Step is, in many ways, all about Emotional Regulation, we'll dedicate one section to deep dive into the topic, covering issues such as coping mechanisms, building confidence and resilience, navigating social challenges, the value of empathy, and positive reinforcement techniques.

Supplements to Support Calming

Supplements like Tyrosine, GABA, L-theanine, and Lactium can also support your child's journey to calmness. At the end of this Step, we'll help you determine if these supplements can be valuable tools for your child.

INFORMATION CENTER

The Impact of ADHD and Gene Expression on the Ability to Calm

Many genes play a role in emotional regulation and, in turn, our ability to adapt and respond calmly and consciously in any given situation.

This will not be surprising to any parent of a child with ADHD who has witnessed massive after-school meltdowns after their child has spent all day masking their true feelings and behaviors to fit the environment. ADHD brains often face unique challenges in reaching and maintaining a state of calm because so much is happening below the surface that disrupts this ability.

One key factor is how easily the body can switch from sympathetic dominance (the fight, flight, freeze, or fawn mode) to parasympathetic dominance (the rest, recuperate, feed, and breed mode). Neurotransmitter production, receptor function, and the efficiency of neurotransmitter transport all influence this critical shift. When these processes are compromised, the ability to calm down after a stressor is significantly hindered.

Another example is bedtime resistance or difficulties settling down in the evening. Many parents report their children with ADHD becoming "wired" just as the rest of the household is winding down. This is not necessarily a conscious choice or a child willfully attempting to counter their bedtime routine. Instead, it is often a reflection of how ADHD impacts neurotransmitter regulation, circadian rhythms, and the ability to engage the parasympathetic system.

With a nod to our RESPOND system found in Chapter 11, when bedtime is not going as planned, take time to Reflect as the first step in managing behavioral challenges. Practice deep breathing as a beginning support for you and your child. Simply take a deep breath through the nose and exhale longer through the mouth—one more time. Now, let's explore how we can better support ourselves and our children in cultivating a core of calm.

Dopamine and ADHD

Let's start this Step by closely examining dopamine. It is a key neurotransmitter involved in the brain's reward, motivation, attention, and executive function pathways, all of which are areas typically affected in individuals with ADHD. Research suggests that ADHD is associated with dysregulation in the dopaminergic system, particularly in places in the brain that are critical for attention, impulse control, and decision-making.

The **COMT** gene encodes an enzyme responsible for breaking down cate-cholamines, including dopamine, epinephrine (also called adrenaline), and nor-epinephrine (noradrenaline), as well as estrogens and certain drugs.

COMT is extremely active in the prefrontal cortex, the area in the brain responsible for cognitive behavior, decision-making, personality expression, learn-ing, addictions (like gambling, screens, video games, the volume of food con-sumed, or shopping), and moderating much of social behavior.

Variations in the COMT gene influence the activity of the enzyme responsible for breaking down dopamine, epinephrine, and norepinephrine. Dopamine plays a critical role in attention, mood regulation, and the ability to stay calm and focused. However, imbalances can also heighten sensitivity to stress and anxiety. Epinephrine and norepinephrine are key components of the body's natural stress response, helping regulate reactions to challenges and threats.

When normal (green), this SNP breaks down dopamine, epinephrine, and norepinephrine faster. These individuals will have reduced dopamine levels and low epinephrine and norepinephrine levels. If the COMT SNP is variant (red), then dopamine will not easily break down and, like epinephrine and norepineph-rine, will be elevated.

In other words, both gene codings (normal and variant) have benefits and challenges. It would be ideal to have plentiful amounts of dopamine in the brain and for messages to easily reach the next neuron. However, we would also love to optimally break down epinephrine and norepinephrine so our stress levels would decrease appropriately when the need for them has passed. What is best with the COMT gene is when it is neither homozygous variant (red) nor homozygous normal (green) but rather heterozygous (yellow, having received the normal cod-ing from one parent and the variant coding from the other). In other words, a Goldilocks position of not too much and not too little.

Importantly, this example highlights that ADHD symptoms are not always tied to "variant" genes; all three versions (green, yellow, and red) may be beneficial depending on the gene and context.

Dopamine and ADHD are frequently discussed in popular media, often implying that simply having enough dopamine could prevent ADHD. However, the story doesn't end with dopamine production and breakdown. For dopamine to have its intended effect, its message must not only be sent across the synapse to the next cell but also successfully received by dopamine receptors in the postsynaptic cell.

Additionally, dopamine can bind to specific receptors on the presynaptic neuron, triggering a negative feedback loop that regulates dopamine release (more on this in the Medical and Alternative Treatments chapter).

This means it's essential to consider both the amount of dopamine present in the brain and how effectively the dopamine receptors—proteins designed to receive and process these signals—are functioning.

To understand this, we turn to another SNP, **DRD2**, which primarily encodes the dopamine receptor D2, a critical component in receiving dopamine signals in the brain. Depending on the genetic coding of this SNP, dopamine receptors may function at near-optimal efficiency (green), around 50% efficiency (yellow), or at significantly reduced efficiency (red). These variations influence how well dopamine signals are transmitted and processed, contributing to differences in focus, motivation, and behavior.

In addition, consider what happens if, regardless of coding, your child's dopamine receptors are inflamed (more on this in Step Six – Inflammation) and unable to receive the message. Or, if your child is under significant stress and experiencing elevated or dysregulated levels of stress hormones like cortisol, this can further impair dopamine signaling. Again, stress and inflammation are potent disruptors that can alter gene expression, effectively causing up to 90% of genes to behave as if they are variant.

In scenarios like this, it's akin to a receiver in a football game who misses the ball—the message doesn't get through. When dopamine signaling is impaired—whether due to reduced dopamine levels, receptor inefficiency, or external factors like stress and inflammation—it can contribute to symptoms such as inattention, impulsivity, and hyperactivity. This is one reason many ADHD medications work by enhancing dopamine activity in the brain, improving both the transmission of dopamine signals and receptor function (explored further in the Medical and Alternative Treatment chapter).

To understand a more complete picture of dopamine, another relevant SNP is **DAT1** (also known as **SLC6A3**). This gene encodes a dopamine transporter protein responsible for regulating dopamine levels in the brain. It facilitates the reuptake of dopamine from the synaptic cleft (the space between neurons) back into the presynaptic neuron for recycling, as a negative feedback mechanism (telling the cell not to make or make more dopamine) or breakdown, reducing the concentration of dopamine in the extracellular space.

In simpler terms, think of it as a "cleanup system" that prevents dopamine from lingering too long in the communication pathway, ensuring the brain can reset and maintain balance. This process directly influences dopamine availability in key brain regions, such as the prefrontal cortex and striatum, which are critical for focus, motivation, and impulse control.

Variants of the receptor SNPs (DRD2 and DAT1) can result in less efficient dopamine reuptake and transportation, reducing dopaminergic activity. This imbalance has been associated with conditions like ADHD, where insufficient dopamine signaling can impact attention and self-regulation.

SNP Peek - Calm Genes

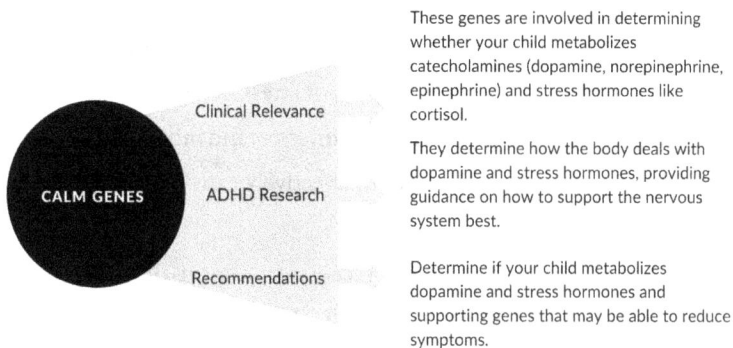

These genes are involved in determining whether your child metabolizes catecholamines (dopamine, norepinephrine, epinephrine) and stress hormones like cortisol.

Clinical Relevance

CALM GENES   ADHD Research

They determine how the body deals with dopamine and stress hormones, providing guidance on how to support the nervous system best.

Recommendations

Determine if your child metabolizes dopamine and stress hormones and supporting genes that may be able to reduce symptoms.

Now, let's put this Core Step's gene information together. By examining the COMT gene, responsible for breaking down dopamine, alongside DRD2 and DAT1, the dopamine receptors genes, we gain insight into how your child metabolizes dopamine and stress hormones like epinephrine and norepinephrine. This provides valuable clues about their ability to focus, maintain attention, and regulate impulses.

The "Worrier" Combination

I (Alicia) am homozygous for the variant (red) of the COMT gene, meaning my COMT enzyme doesn't easily break down dopamine. On the plus side, this higher dopamine level can lead to fewer addictive behaviors and reduced food cravings. It also makes me passionate and enthusiastic about things I love.

However, this variant comes with challenges. Since my COMT gene also struggles to break down stress hormones like epinephrine and norepinephrine, I'm more prone to anxiety and obsessive-compulsive tendencies—earning me the nickname "worrier" in the epigenetics world. This heightened presence of stress hormones can also make me reactive. My kids often tease me about having "no filter" or jumping to respond before others have finished speaking.

The good news is that understanding my genetic tendencies has helped me recognize and manage these behaviors. By slowing down and being more present, I can regulate my reactions and channel my energy more effectively. This deeper self-awareness has made me a more compassionate mom and allowed me to forgive myself for moments when high dopamine and stress hormones likely fueled less-than-ideal parenting decisions.

For a child with ADHD, the "worrier" gene combination can manifest in several ways:

- **Heightened Anxiety and Sensitivity**: Difficulty calming down in stressful situations due to a struggle to break down stress hormones. They may appear easily overwhelmed or worry excessively.

- **Overthinking and Difficulty Letting Go**: Tendency to replay situations or focus excessively on perceived mistakes, which can sometimes lead to meltdowns.

- **Obsessive or Compulsive Tendencies**: Fixating on specific tasks or routines to cope with stress, such as needing things "just so."

- **Impulsive Responses and Reactivity**: Blurting out answers or interrupting conversations due to a racing mind.

- **Difficulty Focusing Under Pressure**: Elevated stress hormones may impair their ability to stay attentive in high-pressure environments.

Despite these challenges, "worrier" children often demonstrate profound strengths, including empathy, curiosity, and passion for their interests. With guidance, their heightened sensitivity can foster creative problem-solving and meaningful connections.

The "Warrior" Combination

Let's now examine the other side of the COMT gene. Brenda's daughter, Rachel, is homozygous for this gene's "normal" coding, meaning her COMT enzyme efficiently and consistently breaks down dopamine. While this might seem advantageous, combined with other gene codings often associated with ADHD, such heightened COMT activity can lower dopamine levels in key brain regions like the prefrontal cortex. This can increase the likelihood of behaviors aimed at boosting dopamine, such as food cravings, attention-seeking, or impulsivity—all of which provide quick dopamine bursts.

On the positive side, Rachel's efficient dopamine breakdown allows her to effectively manage stress hormones like epinephrine and norepinephrine, helping her regulate stress easily. This balance makes her a classic example of the "warrior" type—someone who persists with determination, resilience, and grit.

Rachel's genetic profile also includes a variant for the DAT1 gene, which reduces dopamine reuptake efficiency. This dual challenge—quick dopamine breakdown by COMT and reduced reuptake by DAT1—makes it harder to maintain adequate dopamine levels in the prefrontal cortex, which are crucial for focus, attention, and impulse control.

Given this combination, Rachel's brain requires extra support to maintain optimal dopamine levels. Targeted nutritional strategies—such as supplements like tyrosine, which supports dopamine synthesis—and possibly medication can be highly effective (see Chapter 13 for details).

For a child with ADHD, the "warrior" gene combination may show up as:

- **Difficulty Sustaining Motivation**: Excelling under pressure but struggling with tasks lacking immediate rewards or stimulation.

- **Dopamine-Seeking Behaviors**: Engaging in activities like eating sugary snacks, playing video games, or taking risks to gain quick dopamine boosts.

- **Rigidity in Focus**: Relentless determination that can make them inflexible or overly fixated on specific outcomes.

- **Exceptional Resilience**: Bouncing back quickly from setbacks and demonstrating grit in the face of challenges.

- **Heightened Focus Under Pressure**: Thriving in high-stakes situations where adrenaline enhances concentration and performance.

- Better Emotional Regulation: Thanks to efficient breakdown of stress hormones, they may display a greater tolerance for frustration than their peers.

Dopamine-Seeking Behavior

Whether your child leans more toward the "worrier" or "warrior" genetic profile, each combination offers challenges and strengths and helps determine how more or less aggressively your child seeks dopamine hits. Dopamine, often referred to as the brain's "feel-good" neurotransmitter, plays a critical role in motivation, attention, and reward.

If dopamine levels are low due to insufficient production, impaired dopamine receptors, or overly rapid breakdown, your child's brain will naturally push them to seek out behaviors that elevate dopamine. These might include eating sugary snacks, playing video games, scratching at a sore, or instigating conflict to get a "rise" out of a sibling, parent, or teacher. Suppose your child is deeply engaged in an activity that provides a steady stream of dopamine (e.g., building a Lego masterpiece or playing a favorite video game). In that case, they may become upset, frustrated, or even angry when asked to stop. This is because the dopamine boost they were enjoying is suddenly cut off, leaving them feeling deprived and dysregulated.

At the same time, an imbalance in dopamine—whether too little or too much—can disrupt a child's ability to remain calm. When dopamine levels are too low, the brain struggles to stay engaged and motivated, leading to restlessness, irritability, and frustration. Conversely, when dopamine levels are too high, they can trigger hyperactivity, impulsivity, and even difficulty relaxing or falling asleep. This fine balance helps explain why behaviors aimed at boosting dopamine can often swing a child between states of excitement and dysregulation.

While the term is not scientific, describing children with these dopamine dynamics as "tiny dopamine-seeking missiles" can help us understand their biological drive for activities—positive or negative—that offer instant gratification or immediate reward. This metaphor illustrates their brain's natural tendency to seek dopamine-boosting experiences to regulate their emotional and mental state.

As Dr. Kendall-Reed often emphasizes, understanding DNA validates one's physiological responses and emotions while empowering you to make meaningful changes that support one's health and well-being. Recognizing the role of dopamine in your child's behaviors can guide you toward strategies that balance dopamine naturally, such as incorporating physical activity, creating predictable routines, and offering structured opportunities for dopamine boosts in healthy, productive ways.

In other words, it's crucial to understand both a) how genes interact with each other and b) why this interplay matters. It's not as simple as testing a single gene and concluding, "You break down dopamine well" or "You don't." Instead, you need a more comprehensive view—examining not just dopamine production and breakdown but also whether a neurotransmitter's signal is effectively reaching its destination and how it interacts with other neurotransmitters.

Importantly, dopamine-related genes don't work in isolation. Their expression and effectiveness are also influenced by their interactions with genes governing detoxification, sleep, inflammation, and metabolism. This interconnectedness reminds us to view the body as a whole system rather than focusing on isolated processes. The word "holistic" captures this broader perspective, where understanding one collection of genes—such as those linked to neurotransmitters—means considering how they interact with and are influenced by all relevant systems.

To add to that mix, several other categories of genes are involved in calming, two of which we'll cover next: genes that impact serotonin production and stress.

Serotonin and Stress Response Genes

Serotonin is a key neurotransmitter involved in mood, sleep, and emotional regulation. Here, we focus on its critical role in mood stability and sleep patterns. Genes such as **TPH2** (which facilitates serotonin synthesis) and **MAOA** (responsible for breaking down serotonin, dopamine, epinephrine, and norepinephrine) significantly influence neurotransmitter availability in the brain. MAOA functions similarly to COMT, but with notable differences: being variant for MAOA slows the breakdown of serotonin and dopamine, which may reduce symptoms of depression and increase motivation. However, faster clearance of epinephrine and norepinephrine in those with normal MAOA coding can help decrease anxiety and panic disorders. This illustrates how multiple genes interact to influence ADHD-related traits.

Another important stress response gene is **FKBP5**. This gene influences how our bodies respond to pressure or distress, affecting cortisol levels and overall stress management. It influences the negative feedback loop of the Hypothalamic-Pituitary-Adrenal (HPA) axis (i.e., how the brain and adrenal glands communicate) and can foster prolonged cortisol production or dysregulation.

Children with certain variations in this gene might have a heightened stress response and more easily stay stuck in fight-or-flight mode, making it harder to stay calm in challenging situations. As anyone with a homozygous variant for FKBP5 will attest (Here, Brenda gets to raise her hand!), being stuck in "stress" is not fun. When a child or parent cannot easily move into parasympathetic mode and calm down, it can be upsetting for all concerned!

Another gene we look at to understand stress responses is the **CRHR1** SNP. This SNP is a receptor that binds corticotropin-releasing hormone (CRH), stimulating the HPA axis and pushing the nervous system to the sympathetic stress side. This action stimulates the pituitary (also within the HPA axis) to release

ACTH, which, in turn, stimulates the adrenals to produce cortisol, adrenaline, and noradrenaline. And, of course, as with all genes, it interacts with other genes, in this case, COMT, DRD2, and MAOA. The variant allele for CRHR1 has increased CRH receptors, which may be the reason it causes increased anxiety and depression. It may also affect the GI tract and cause bloating, gas, or irregular bowel movements.

In this section, we'll examine one additional gene, **GAD1**. This gene plays a crucial role in the production of gamma-aminobutyric acid (GABA), a neurotransmitter that helps calm the nervous system. This gene, too, can impact how well a child relaxes and manages stress.

Variants in the GAD1 gene can affect how efficiently the body converts glutamate, an excitatory neurotransmitter, into GABA, a calming neurotransmitter that reduces neural activity, promotes relaxation, reduces anxiety, and plays a role in sleep regulation. An excess of glutamate and insufficient conversion to GABA can lead to overstimulation, making it harder for a child to relax and manage stress.

The issue with excess glutamate is another reason why it's crucial to continually cycle back to Step One – Eat and be mindful of food ingredients, particularly additives like MSG (monosodium glutamate), which can increase glutamate levels in the brain. Checking labels and avoiding foods with hidden MSG may help reduce overstimulation and support a calmer nervous system.

I (Alicia) met someone who was getting headaches in response to food containing glutamate. After investigating, he realized that the food contained MSG, which was the root cause of the problem. His genetics show that he is a variant for GAD1. Eliminating his exposure to MSG eliminated the headaches.

I (Alicia) was born and grew up in Mexico City. In Mexican culture, using Knorr Suiza (chicken bouillon) in cooking is the norm. Knorr Suiza contains MSG, and I don't metabolize it (I, too, am variant for GAD1). Not only do I have high levels of dopamine, epinephrine, and norepinephrine, but it is also hard to feel calm when I consume MSG. This response to glutamate is one of the primary reasons why, for me, the best way of eating is reading labels, shopping wisely, cooking my meals, and leaving out ingredients I know will be problematic for my well-being.

Understanding these genetic factors helps us appreciate why mindfulness and meditation can be particularly effective in both supporting a child with ADHD's strengths and minimizing some of the situation mismatch limitations. By optimally fueling, fostering sound sleep, promoting joyful movement, and engaging in practices that promote calm and focus (e.g., breathwork and supplement use), we can help balance the impact of these genetic variations.

Mindfulness

Mindfulness is the practice of paying attention to the present moment without judgment. It's about being fully aware of what's happening now, whether it's the sound of birds, your breath, or the taste of an apple. For children with ADHD, mindfulness can be a powerful tool for managing hyperactivity and intrusive thoughts. By focusing on the present, children learn to observe their thoughts and feelings without being overwhelmed, reducing impulsivity and improving focus.

Research shows that mindfulness improves attention, emotional regulation, and impulsivity. It activates brain regions involved in sustaining attention, such as the prefrontal cortex (PFC) and anterior cingulate cortex (ACC). With regular practice, children can strengthen these areas, enhancing focus and self-control. Mindfulness also improves working memory, concentration, and resilience, helping children navigate daily challenges.

Breathwork, Imagery, and Binaural Beats

Mindful breathing is a simple but effective calming exercise that also supports detoxification. Encourage slow, deep breaths, focusing on the sensation of air entering and leaving the body. Breathing in through the nose and exhaling slowly through the mouth activates the relaxation response, reducing stress.

Guided imagery, where your child imagines a peaceful scene like a gentle stream, can help distract from intrusive thoughts and promote calm. Non-Sleep Deep Rest (NSDR), which involves deeply relaxing the body while staying awake, can rejuvenate the mind and body. Body scans, where your child notices sensations from toes to head, increase body awareness and promote relaxation.

Binaural beats are another calming tool that supports sleep and relaxation. Parents can access free binaural beats for their child through platforms like YouTube, which offers a wide variety of tracks specifically designed for focus, relaxation, or sleep. Apps like Insight Timer or Brain.fm also provide free or trial content featuring binaural beats tailored to different needs. Always ensure the chosen content aligns with the desired goal.

Incorporating mindfulness into daily routines doesn't have to be complicated. Start with small practices, like mindful breathing in the morning or guided imagery before bed. Mindful eating—encouraging your child to experience the taste and texture of food—can make mealtime calming. Mindfulness breaks during the day, like focusing on surroundings, can also help reset attention and reduce stress.

Routines

Routines are powerful for managing ADHD, offering predictability and security that reduce anxiety. A morning routine might include visual cues for brushing teeth and getting dressed, while a homework routine could use a checklist with breaks. These tools help children stay on track and reduce the mental load of remembering steps.

Create a visual schedule with colorful charts outlining daily activities. Use pictures to represent each task, making it easier for your child to follow. Timeboxing (i.e., physically setting aside time in the family schedule for tasks) and checklists with specifics (e.g., all the items needed to be done to get ready for school) provide a sense of accomplishment and keep your child on track.

If you need a simple idea of implementing and following through on those routines engagingly, consider purchasing a ready-made magnetic schedule. I (Brenda) have a friend, Elaine Tan Comeau, a mama and former teacher who created an excellent, award-winning family organizational product called Daysies® Daily Schedules (https://www.easydaysies.com/) to help show kids the "shape of the day." Elaine told me, "Visual schedules help children feel safe and confident as they can see and predict what is happening next, improving executive functioning, independence, and cooperation while lessening anxiety." Child psychologists and occupational therapists mention Elaine's changeable and age-appropriate charts as a great support to children with autism, ADHD, or other special needs. They could be a great start to a fun routine for your child.

Flexibility

Flexibility within routines is essential for children with ADHD. While structure provides a framework, it's important to accommodate their dynamic needs. For example, if your child is particularly restless, substitute a quiet activity for something more active. Conversely, if your child is having trouble with a calm activity and has entered dopamine-seeking behavior—continuously swatting at a sibling, picking at their cuticles, back talking or yelling, and looking for a "rise" out of you—it may be you need to switch to an activity that provides positive mini-dopamine hits such as having races to the end of the block with "high fives" after each race.

Maintaining the overall structure while adapting to your child's current state helps prevent power struggles, assists with dopamine regulation, and creates a harmonious environment.

As a parent, modeling routines is crucial. Consistency is key, and your actions set the tone. We had a Thursday family night when our (Brenda's) kids were young. The children contributed a variety of ideas of what we could do together. They wrote the activities on slips of paper, which we folded and put in a jar. Each week, one of the children had their turn to pick a slip, which would be our evening activity.

Along with weekly family time, all five had set bedtime routines (e.g., snack, bath, PJs on, teeth brushed, story time, prayers), and we had weekly activities that all our children, including Rachel, really looked forward to. We also had our children involved in routines other than family night and bedtime by creating visual schedules for some of them or letting them choose the order of their homework tasks or which chores they'd do at our Saturday household clean-up time. This involvement empowered our children, made them more invested in following the routine, and produced five very fun, productive, relational, AND fairly organized adults!

Emotional Regulation

Imagine your child going from zero to meltdown in seconds because their younger sister borrowed their favorite shirt and left it crumpled in the corner. Suddenly, you're dealing with an eruption that rivals Mount Vesuvius. Emotional dysregulation can turn everyday situations into high-stakes drama. As a mom (Brenda) who's been there (and could name the younger sister!), recognizing the warning signs is the first step to managing these emotional roller coasters.

In children with ADHD, emotional dysregulation manifests as quick tempers, mood swings, and frustration. This isn't just a "bad day"—it's often triggered by lifestyle factors like poor sleep, excess sugar, or too much screen time. Neurobiologically, some of the genes we've mentioned—COMT, DRD2, MAOA, and GAD1—affect planning, decision-making, and impulse control, making emotional regulation harder. The prefrontal cortex, responsible for managing emotions, doesn't always communicate well with the amygdala, leading to over-reactions.

Simple tools like deep breathing can help calm your child by activating the parasympathetic nervous system. Teach them to inhale for four counts and exhale for six. Again, binaural beats or guided imagery can also provide relief.

Whether we like it or not, parents play a crucial role in modeling emotional regulation. If you stay calm during stressful moments, your child will likely do the same. I distinctly remember a heated argument with Rachel—then a teenager with Lyme disease and undiagnosed ADHD. After storming off to our bedroom, I vented to my husband, "I feel like being immature and just leaving it unresolved." He said, "You're the parent, her safe place. You can't." So, I took a few deep breaths, reminded myself of my emotional regulation tools, and re-engaged. Sometimes, re-engagement ended well, sometimes not—but I operated from a foundation of unconditional love, knowing that managing emotions for Rachel and myself was a skill learned over time.

Building Confidence and Resilience

Encouraging children to engage in activities where they excel builds resilience and self-esteem. Consider your child's strengths—building intricate Lego structures or being entrepreneurial like Rachel, who started a neighborhood shaved ice stand and saved enough money to go to summer camp. These activities are more than just fun; they allow your child to experience success and build self-esteem. As my husband used to tell Rachel's three older brothers, "Be nice to Rach; it's likely you're going to be working for her someday!"

Social skills training can help children with ADHD navigate peer relationships by teaching them social cues and conflict resolution through role-playing and interactive games. Practicing these at home reinforces positive behaviors.

Sadly, bullying of children with ADHD is common, so teach your child to recognize and report it and practice assertive responses like, "Stop, I don't like that." Note that teasing, too, often seeming to be simply done for fun, can also be emotionally damaging. If family teasing happens, ensure it is done kindly and check in with the "teasee" to ensure they are okay with what is happening.

The Importance of Empathy

Empathy strengthens the parent-child bond. When your child is upset, listen and validate their feelings before offering solutions. Say, "I see you're upset; let's talk about it." This type of communication shows them that their emotions matter. Empathy also transforms discipline—understand what's behind their behavior and guide them toward better choices. This fosters emotional security and trust.

While modeling empathy, remember to have your child repeat statements to you such as, "I see *you* are upset. Do you want to talk about it?" Compassion for yourself is also essential.

Positive Reinforcement Techniques

Positive reinforcement is a powerful way to encourage desired behaviors and boost self-esteem. When you highlight small achievements and link them to immediate rewards, whether extra playtime or praise, you are helping your child grow in seeking dopamine in positive ways. Consistent, fair rewards also help children understand the connection between their actions and positive outcomes.

Supplements For Calming Support

Supplements can help promote calmness and relaxation. As mentioned in Step Three – Sleep, one of our most recommended supplements contains Lactium, a bioactive decapeptide derived from milk. Lactium has been shown to reduce stress and improve sleep quality by modulating the HPA axis and helping to regulate stress hormone levels like cortisol. When combined with L-theanine, this compound supports the nervous system, ensuring signals are "heard" and acted upon.

L-theanine, found in green tea, promotes relaxation and improves focus without causing drowsiness. It increases the production of GABA and serotonin, supporting calmness.

When I (Alicia) first did a gene "reset" with lifestyle and supplement changes (including taking Lactium), within three and a half weeks, I experienced a calmness I'd never felt before. I take one Lactium before bedtime, but I'll take another in the morning if I expect a stressful day. Once, when this supplement was backordered, Brenda noticed how "all over the place" I was and offered me a bottle from her own supply. What a relief (to both of us!) Of all the supplements we suggest, a high-quality Lactium supplement is one we hope your child (and possibly you, too) can try soon.

Gamma-aminobutyric acid is another neurotransmitter that inhibits neural activity, promoting relaxation and reducing anxiety. GABA supplements can help calm the mind and body, making it easier for children with ADHD to manage stress. Since GABA can have difficulty binding to receptors, a support supplement like passionflower can increase GABA uptake.

Where dopamine dysregulation plays a role in ADHD symptoms, maintaining adequate levels of tyrosine—an amino acid that is a precursor of dopamine—can help support dopamine production. With the help of cofactors like iron, zinc, vitamin B6, and other B vitamins, tyrosine is converted into dopamine, a key neurotransmitter for mood, focus, and motivation.

While research is limited, understanding genetic interactions suggests that those with low dopamine may benefit from tyrosine supplementation or foods containing higher amounts of tyrosine, like chicken, turkey, fish, dairy, nuts, seeds, and fermented soy products. Keep in mind that if you are like me (Alicia), where I already have too much dopamine, tyrosine does nothing for me neurotransmitter-wise. Knowing which supplements will benefit your child is one of the true gifts of understanding their genetics.

If your child has a TPH2 gene variant that affects the conversion of tryptophan to 5-HTP (e.g., is homozygous for variant or heterozygous), crucial for serotonin production, supplementation with 5-HTP may help support serotonin levels. The amino acid 5-HTP is a direct precursor to serotonin, making it an effective supplement for supporting mood, sleep, and other serotonin-regulated functions.

Supplement effects can vary significantly between individuals—for example, a supplement that helps most children sleep better might cause your child to wake up during the night. More research is needed to understand the potential of amino acid supplements fully.

In a recent webinar, Dr. Greenblatt shared a case study of a woman with depression caused by an inability to break down proteins into amino acids despite following a clean, whole-food diet. Sometimes, underlying issues like low stomach acid or poor digestion may cause similar challenges.

Supplements can be valuable additions to your child's routine when used in the right combination and dosage. That's why understanding their mechanisms is crucial. Begin by examining how your child's stress response genes interact, then consult a healthcare professional to determine appropriate dosages based on your child's size, weight, and unique genetic profile.

TRAVELER ASSISTANCE

One remarkable benefit of an ADHD brain is its ability to engage deeply with interesting and exciting activities. When channeled correctly, this hyperfocus can be a great asset. Mindfulness and structured routines help harness this ability, turning it into a tool for calmness and productivity. When your child learns to direct their focus mindfully, they can achieve impressive concentration and creativity. This unique strength can be nurtured through consistent practice, leading to better emotional regulation, a stronger sense of control, and positively fostered dopamine.

Mindfulness and routines aren't just about managing symptoms; they empower your child. I (Brenda) recall when Rachel was in her tree-climbing phase. She'd been playing with her siblings near our home and fell from a branch into prickly bushes, leaving her with deep scratches on her back. While she wasn't seriously injured, she was anxious and in discomfort. I had been using "tapping" (e.g., Emotional Freedom Technique) to calm my own anxious thoughts, so I taught it to Rachel to help with her pain and anxiety as she healed. She quickly became a pro at tapping, running to her room several times daily to use this simple technique to relieve the pain and irritation.

Watch instructional videos on The Tapping Solution YouTube channel for easy tapping guidelines.

REST STOP

Time for parents to take a break and digest information! Take 10 minutes of calm to Rest with the following questions:

1. **Assess Your Own Calming Strategies**: How do you model calmness in your daily life? Are there moments when your emotional state might contribute to your child's dysregulation? Reflect on areas where you might need to focus on your own calming strategies to support your child better.

2. **Balance Structure and Flexibility**: Think about the level of structure versus flexibility in your child's daily routine. Is there a balance between providing enough predictability to feel safe and calm while also allowing for moments of spontaneity and choice? How could adjusting this balance help in supporting your child's self-regulation?

Next, Stop for 10 minutes of quiet (sitting or slowly walking). Keep your mind as clear and open as possible, and just listen. Jot down or tell Siri to "make a note" of any responses that may arise. Because you've taken time to ponder calmly and quietly, these responses will most likely be less off-the-cuff and from a deeper level. They can give you clues as to the reasons behind your answers! Those clues, in turn, will reveal potential problematic thinking and can provide great direction on moving forward with the recommendations in this Step that would be the easiest to implement or fit best for your family!

A parent's reaction to their child's behavior is crucial in shaping their emotional and behavioral development. Key principles include:

- **Self-Regulation for Parents:** We encourage you to understand and manage your emotional responses before addressing your child's behavior. This is rooted in the belief that children often mirror their parents' emotional states. Taking this step will require both your own emotional work and your ability to self-regulate quickly in instances when your child cannot.

- **Empathy and Validation:** Instead of reacting impulsively or punitively, it is important to empathize with your child's experience and validate their feelings. For instance, acknowledging frustration or anger without immediately imposing discipline.

- **Reframing Behavior:** Challenging behaviors should, for the most part, be seen not as defiance but as signals of unmet needs, developmental challenges, or lagging skills. Addressing the underlying causes rather than just the outward behavior improves outcomes.

We will expand on our RESPOND Framework later, but consider what could happen if you mindfully responded before reacting.

ROADWORK

This Step's Roadwork includes instructions for you and your child to create a Mindfulness Jar, a simple, fun, and effective way to practice mindfulness.

Create Your Own Mindfulness Jar

Materials:

- A clear jar with a lid

- Water

- Colored sand or fine beads

- Food coloring (optional)

Directions:

1. **Fill the Jar:** Fill the jar with water, leaving some space at the top.

2. **Add Sand or Beads:** Add a few spoonfuls of sand or fine beads to the jar. For extra visual appeal, add a drop of food coloring.

3. **Seal the Lid:** Ensure the lid is tightly sealed to prevent leaks.

4. **Shake and Observe:** Shake the jar and watch the sand or beads swirl and settle. Encourage your child to focus on the movement of the sand and beads as they settle, using this as a calming visual aid.

Optional:

A small amount of glycerin or clear dish soap can be added to the water to slow down the movement of sand or beads, creating a more prolonged and calming effect as they settle.

This mindfulness jar can be helpful during moments of stress or overwhelm. It provides a visual focus that promotes calmness.

SOUVENIR

For this Step's souvenir, we offer a method for creating rhythmic discipline in your home based on Effective Parenting techniques centered around four principles: rhythm, polarities, transitions, and clear expectations. First, however, we'll emphasize the importance of implementing these principles. This will help create a calmer household, with fewer struggles over routines and more evident roles for everyone. It will also foster a sense of hope and motivation for parents.

A central aspect of Effective Parenting's approach, rhythmic discipline, emphasizes creating harmony in the home through structure and consistency.

- **Rhythm:** Establishing predictable daily routines, like consistent mealtimes, bedtime rituals, and homework schedules, to provide children with a sense of stability and security.

- **Polarities:** Recognizing and balancing opposites in a child's experience—such as activity and rest, freedom, and boundaries. For example, allowing a period of free play after structured learning time to encourage balance (this also ties in with Dr. Melillo's work on hemispheric balance).

- **Transitions:** Supporting children through changes (e.g., shifting from playtime to dinner) by providing warnings, clear cues, or rituals. For example, a countdown or a song to signal the end of an activity.

- **Clear Expectations:** Setting clear, age-appropriate rules and consistently enforcing them. This approach avoids ambiguity and helps children understand boundaries without feeling overly controlled.

Techniques

You'll find reminders of these tools scattered throughout our book, but here they're listed as great tools to implement in your household to foster emotional intelligence and cooperation:

- **Use of Storytelling:** Use stories to help you and your child understand emotions and behavior in a non-confrontational way.

- **Family Meetings:** Hold regular check-ins to allow family members to express their thoughts and feelings and collaborate on solving problems.

- **Positive Reinforcement:** Celebrate small successes to encourage desirable behavior and strengthen the parent-child bond.

I (Alicia) remember that as a child, when my mom called the family together for a meal, she would get upset if we took extra time to get to the table—a pattern modeled to her when she was growing up. These abrupt transitions were tough for me, and often, a meal would begin with some members almost at odds with each other.

These days, I have asked my husband to give me a 5 to 10-minute warning before dinner so I can complete whatever I am doing. It makes sense. Otherwise, if I'm late to the table, frustration might ensue, and when I get downstairs, like Goldilocks and the Three Bears, I will further complicate the situation by eating cold soup!

Children with ADHD often love structure, and by creating a rhythmic discipline, you'll enjoy a more peaceful environment.

Before we move on, here is a little note on a term we use in our book, "age-appropriate." As mentioned, children with ADHD can experience developmental delays—an often-cited figure is 3-5 years—particularly in areas related to executive functioning (e.g., impulse control, organization, planning, emotional regulation). That means age-appropriate guidelines or expectations will mean different things for a neurotypical 8-year-old vs. an 8-year-old with ADHD.

Because of their particular genetics, someone with ADHD may never find certain activities to be easy, so setting clear expectations, finding an organizational system, setting routines in place, and providing planning assistance in a way that works with that brain is going to be the most effective way to deal with it.

As one of our friends, a mom with ADHD, parenting a child with ADHD reminded us, working with your child in a way that respects the way they function requires letting go of the expectation that ADHD brains *should* be able to do what neurotypical brains can do.

For example, she mentioned that every day after school, her son's socks would end up on the floor somewhere, most often in the living room, sometimes in her bedroom, the bathroom, or the kitchen. She got SO tired of it, especially since each pair required A LOT of work on her part to get her son to pick them up. So she put a basket for his dirty socks on the shoe rack by the front door (point of performance where he takes off his shoes), and she doesn't think she has seen a single dirty sock on the floor since then. Note taken (and more on point of performance to come)!

Next up is inflammation and its role in ADHD symptoms.

Chapter 9

Core Step Six – Inflammation

"Inflammation is not the fire, it is the firetruck. Treat the causes, not the symptom."

— Dr. Mark Hyman, author of The Blood Sugar Solution
10-Day Detox Diet

SUMMARY - Travel Size Version

With Suzanne, an 8-year-old with ADHD, her parents noticed that her propensity to symptoms such as ruminating or intrusive thoughts seemed to flare up whenever she ate certain foods or was under stress. After consulting with a healthcare provider, they discovered that Suzanne had higher levels of inflammatory markers. By making simple changes like switching to an anti-inflammatory diet and incorporating regular, gentle physical activity, Suzanne's parents saw a significant improvement in her thinking patterns and overall well-being.

They also tried some additional practical methods, like using castor oil packs and giving her magnesium supplements before bed. These methods helped reduce Suzanne's inflammation and made her feel calmer and more focused.

Inflammation is like your body's alarm system. When something isn't right—like an infection or an injury—your body calls for help. This call brings in immune cells to fight off the invaders and start the healing process. However, when this alarm system stays on for too long, it can cause problems, especially for children with ADHD. Think of it like a fire alarm that never stops ringing.

Inflammation Genes

Chronic inflammation, a condition that can be hard to diagnose or determine, can cause a variety of issues, including making ADHD's challenging symptoms worse. Therefore, as usual, we will break down the complex science of inflammation genes and ADHD into bite-sized, easy-to-digest pieces.

Contributing Factors to Inflammation

Not only do specific genes impact our body's ability to foster and control inflammation, but many other lifestyle choices, such as diet, movement, and sleep, also influence the degree of inflammation one experiences. Here, we help you understand these factors and give insight into accounting for them.

Managing Inflammation

Next, we will cover some practical steps you can take at home to help manage inflammation, including a couple of different types of hydrotherapy.

Supplements for Inflammation

Supplements can also be crucial in managing inflammation. We'll examine minerals, antioxidants, and other supplements that have anti-inflammatory properties and can support overall brain health.

Castor Oil Packs

We'll wrap up this Step by sharing information on castor oil packs, one of our favorite tools for dealing with inflammation and detoxification.

INFORMATION CENTER

It's a typical Tuesday evening, and you've just finished dinner. As you clear the table, you notice your child scratching at their skin and complaining about an ache in their joints. Or perhaps before bed, they're unusually irritable and restless. You've heard inflammation might play a role in ADHD, but 1) what does that even mean, and 2) what would that look like in your child's day-to-day life?

The Role of Inflammation in Physiological Responses

Let's start by giving a simple example of inflammation and how it looks. If you forcefully bang your shin on the sharp corner of a bed, it will get red and hot.

Inflammation sets in, and there is pain. However, inflammation is not as easy to recognize when it is internal. Acute inflammation can be simpler to notice, but chronic inflammation may even be "silent" because we get used to it in the long term.

Inflammation is the body's natural response to injury or infection. Think of it as your body's internal alarm system. When something goes wrong, like an injury or an invasion by bacteria, your body sends a distress signal. This signal ramps up the production of immune cells and other substances to fight off the invaders and start the healing process. However, when this response becomes disorganized, erratic, or poorly functioning and becomes chronic, it can lead to a host of issues, particularly for children with ADHD.

Inflammation Genes

Let's start by examining the science behind inflammation and its impact on ADHD. Two key genes, **IL6** and **TNF-α**, significantly regulate inflammatory responses. The IL6 gene, specifically the IL6 polymorphism, has been associated with elevated levels of the pro-inflammatory cytokine interleukin-6 (IL-6). This cytokine is like the body's smoke or fire alarm, alerting the immune system to respond to threats. Elevated IL-6 levels have been linked as a contributing factor to various inflammatory conditions, including ADHD.

These two SNPs—IL6 and TNF-α—are associated with altered expression of cytokines, inflammatory molecules that are part of the body's immune response. Cytokines have also been reported in scientific research to play a pivotal role in dopaminergic pathways in the brain, which are also implicated in ADHD. Accordingly, it is conceivable that alterations in pro-inflammatory and anti-inflammatory cytokines may be influential in how inflammation could contribute to ADHD symptoms.

In particular, IL-6 has been reported to cause neurotransmission changes similar to those seen in ADHD, such as increased norepinephrine and reduced dopamine levels. How does this gene interact with the COMT, DRD2, and DAT1 genes? When the receptors are inflamed, message transmission will likely be impaired.

SNP Peek - Inflammation Genes

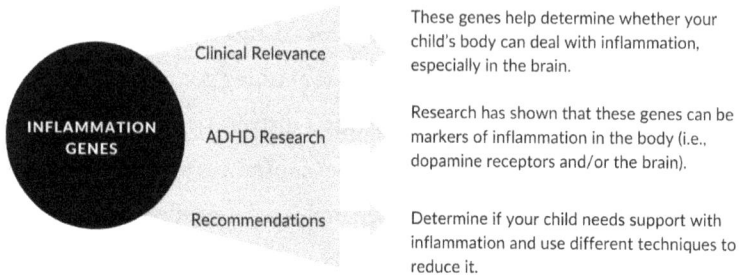

INFLAMMATION GENES

Clinical Relevance — These genes help determine whether your child's body can deal with inflammation, especially in the brain.

ADHD Research — Research has shown that these genes can be markers of inflammation in the body (i.e., dopamine receptors and/or the brain).

Recommendations — Determine if your child needs support with inflammation and use different techniques to reduce it.

If receptors within the synapses are inflamed, dopamine will not reach the next neuron or return to the presynaptic neuron. It will accumulate outside cells and eventually be metabolized in the adrenal glands to norepinephrine. So, if we look at inflammation in relation to ADHD, not only will dopamine not be able to attach correctly to another receptor, but stress levels could increase.

Contributing Factors to Inflammation

Note, too, that an inflammatory response doesn't just stay in one part of the body—it has far-reaching effects on various physiological processes, including gut health, joint health, and brain function. In the gut, chronic inflammation can disrupt the balance of beneficial bacteria, leading to digestive issues that can further impact behavior and mood. You might notice that certain foods seem to trigger bouts of irritability or hyperactivity in your child, which could be a sign of underlying inflammation.

Refer to Step One – Eat, where we discussed that carbohydrates can be inflammatory in the GI tract. That is often where we first notice inflammation, starting with the stomach or the small intestine. The inflammation can be due to undigested food or, if we are sensitive to carbohydrates, having too many at a meal or snack—popcorn, anyone? Something that I (Alicia) always have handy is digestive enzymes. They are easy to take and ease bloating and gas when inflammation hits the gut.

Even if inflammation is first noticed in the GI tract, however, that doesn't mean it is contained there. Inflammation can also cause pain and stiffness in the joints, making it harder for your child to engage in physical activities that are crucial for managing ADHD symptoms.

We remember one of our clients, Liz, being concerned because she couldn't wear her engagement ring due to inflammation in her fingers. As we went through decreasing inflammation, first by optimizing macronutrients (see Step One – Eat), the inflammation subsided quickly, and she was thrilled about it. She made our day with this message: "I'm really loving the program, and TODAY I got my engagement ring on, and my smaller wedding band went on too! First time in months."

As often happens for people new to the epigenetic journey, our client was concerned about what she could see: her swollen fingers. Meanwhile, we were thinking in more holistic terms. If there is inflammation in her fingers, most likely, there is inflammation in other places in the body. This comprehensive approach is "the magic" of reducing systemic inflammation and allowing other body parts to work optimally.

Inflammation can be especially harmful to the brain. Neuroinflammation— or inflammation within the brain—can disrupt neurotransmitter function and worsen ADHD symptoms. Elevated levels of inflammatory markers like IL-6 and TNF-α have been found in children with ADHD, suggesting a connection between inflammation and the severity of ADHD symptoms. Inflammation in the brain can affect areas responsible for attention, impulse control, and emotional regulation, making it even more challenging for your child to manage their symptoms. As mentioned, inflammation may also disrupt dopaminergic metabolism, receptors, and other areas like sleep.

The impact of inflammation on a child with ADHD can be profound, manifesting as both chronic and acute responses. Chronic inflammation is like a slow-burning fire that never entirely goes out, constantly smoldering and causing damage over time. It can lead to persistent symptoms such as mood swings, fatigue, and difficulty concentrating.

Acute inflammation is like a sudden flare-up, often in response to a specific trigger like an infection or injury. These flare-ups can cause sudden worsening of ADHD symptoms, making it harder for your child to cope with everyday tasks.

Many factors can contribute to inflammation, including diet, stress, and environmental toxins. Foods high in sugar and processed ingredients can trigger inflammatory responses, as can, in some people, an intake of nightshade vegetables (e.g., potatoes, eggplant, tomatoes, peppers). A diet rich in anti-inflammatory foods like vegetables (other than nightshades), fruit, and omega-3 fatty acids can often mitigate these effects.

Stress is another major contributor to inflammation. When your child is stressed, their body produces cortisol, which can promote inflammation if levels remain elevated for too long. Environmental toxins, such as those found in air pollution and certain household products, can also trigger inflammatory responses, further complicating the management of ADHD symptoms.

Managing Inflammation

Though inflammation is a relatively complex physiological process, managing inflammation doesn't have to be overwhelming. There are several simple, practical methods that you can incorporate into your daily routine to help reduce inflammation and support your child's overall health.

One effective method is the use of previously mentioned castor oil packs. Castor oil has been used for centuries for its anti-inflammatory properties. Though more robust scientific research is needed to confirm some of the traditionally believed benefits, they are thought to improve the flow of lymphatic fluid, helping transport nutrients to cells more efficiently while aiding in removing waste products and toxins from the body.

Additionally, castor oil packs may enhance circulation, reduce inflammation, and promote relaxation by stimulating the parasympathetic nervous system. Some studies suggest they can support liver health and improve digestion by promoting gentle, natural detoxification. Castor oil packs can be a bit of work to make and use, but they are definitely worth the effort. You'll find complete instructions in this Step's Traveler Assistance.

Icing and cold showers are other effective methods for managing inflammation. Applying ice packs to inflamed areas can help reduce swelling and alleviate pain. Cold showers, though potentially unpleasant, can stimulate circulation and reduce inflammation. Start with short bursts of cold water at the end of a warm shower to help your child acclimate to the temperature change. (Brenda here ... while I value the use of cold water with inflammation, I'm not a big fan of cold showers, so when we say short, we mean short! To start, try 10-30 seconds.)

Hydrotherapy, which involves alternating between hot and cold water, can also be beneficial. This practice stimulates blood flow and helps reduce inflammation. You can incorporate hydrotherapy by having your child alternate between warm and cold compresses or using a shower head that allows for easy temperature adjustments.

Supplements for Inflammation

Supplements, too, can be crucial in managing inflammation. Magnesium, for instance, is known for its anti-inflammatory properties and can help reduce muscle tension and promote relaxation.

Resveratrol, a compound found in grapes and berries, has anti-inflammatory and antioxidant properties. It can help reduce inflammation and support overall brain health.

Two supplements we discussed in Step Four – Detox, N-acetylcysteine (NAC) and glutathione, can also help with inflammation. NAC is a powerful supplement that supports the production of glutathione, a potent antioxidant that helps detoxify the body and reduce inflammation. Liposomal glutathione is a bioavailable form of glutathione that can provide additional support in reducing oxidative stress and inflammation.

After consulting with a healthcare provider, if indicated, including these supplements in your child's daily routine can provide significant benefits in managing inflammation and supporting their overall well-being.

TRAVELER ASSISTANCE

We've previously given simple guidance on how to make and use a castor oil pack. For this Traveler Assistance, we'll provide more complete directions.

Castor Oil Packs

Castor oil packs have a long history of traditional use. While the castor bean is known primarily for its laxative properties, it is also often used in pack form, where the oil is absorbed into lymphatic circulation to provide soothing and cleansing benefits. In this form, castor oil stimulates immune system functioning, decreases inflammation, relaxes muscles, and tonifies and detoxifies internal organs.

Castor oil packs have many applications and can be used for a range of issues, such as:

- Inflammation

- Congestion

- Constipation

- Liver, kidney, and pelvic disorders

- Arthritis

- General detoxification

Directions:

Castor oil packs should not be used when pregnant, breastfeeding, on broken skin, or during heavy menstrual flow. Castor oil should never be taken internally.

The packs are made of cotton or wool flannel (an old flannel sheet will do), folded four-ply (roughly 8" x 8"), and saturated with cold-pressed castor oil (the cloth should be saturated but not dripping).

Castor oil should be purchased as certified organic. It will be very thick and sticky. The oil-saturated flannel is placed directly on the skin and covered with plastic, such as a plastic bag or wrap. Heat from a hot water bottle or heating pad is then applied over the pack. A blanket or towel can be placed over the heat source to keep everything in place. Leave the pack on for 45-60 minutes at a time.

A castor oil pack can be placed on the following body regions:

- The upper right quadrant of the abdomen to stimulate and detoxify the liver.

- Inflamed and swollen joints, bursitis, and muscle strains.

- The abdomen to relieve constipation and other digestive disorders.

- The lower abdomen in cases of menstrual irregularities and uterine/ovarian cysts.

The flannel can be stored in a plastic bag and used over again. Add extra castor oil as needed and replace the pack when it begins to discolor or becomes odorous (usually after several months). After the treatment, if required, you can clean your skin with two teaspoons of baking soda dissolved in one quart of water.

For optimal results, it is generally recommended that a castor oil pack be used for a minimum of four consecutive days a week for a minimum of 4-6 weeks (or up to several months). Using the pack daily, however, will produce the most beneficial results.

After the initial six-week period, here are guidelines for further use:

General Maintenance

- **Frequency:** 1-2 times per week.

- **Purpose:** Supports ongoing detoxification, maintains lymphatic flow, and promotes general wellness.

- **Use Case:** Ideal for individuals without acute symptoms who want to sustain the benefits of detoxification and relaxation.

For Inflammation

- **Frequency:** 3-4 times per week or as needed during flare-ups.

- **Use Case:** To reduce localized swelling and discomfort, focus on areas of pain or inflammation, such as joints, muscles, or the abdomen.

- **Duration:** Continue until symptoms subside, then transition to a maintenance schedule.

For Digestive Troubles
- **Frequency:** 3-5 times per week during periods of digestive distress (e.g., bloating, constipation, IBS).

- **Use Case:** Apply over the abdomen to stimulate digestion, improve bowel movements, and reduce inflammation in the gut.

- **Duration:** Adjust based on improvements, tapering off to 1-2 times per week once digestion normalizes.

For Stress and Relaxation
- **Frequency:** As needed or 2-3 times per week during periods of heightened stress.

- **Use Case:** Castor oil packs can stimulate the parasympathetic nervous system, so they can be applied before bedtime to promote relaxation and better sleep.

- **Duration:** Can be used ongoing, especially during stressful periods.

For Chronic Conditions
- **Frequency:** 3-4 times per week for chronic conditions like autoimmune diseases or recurring inflammation.

- **Use Case:** Regular use can help manage symptoms by reducing systemic inflammation and supporting liver detoxification.

- **Duration:** Discuss with a healthcare provider for personalized recommendations.

Key Notes for Long-Term Use
- **Listen to Your Body:** Adjust frequency and duration based on your feelings and any symptoms you are addressing.

- **Consistency Matters:** Even if less frequent, regular use helps maintain the benefits over time.

- **Consult a Professional:** If symptoms persist or worsen, seek guidance from a healthcare provider.

This flexible approach allows castor oil packs to remain a sustainable part of a wellness routine while effectively addressing specific needs.

In my (Brenda) household, when our children were growing up and super active, we had several COPs on the go at a time. We'd store them in ziplock bags and add castor oil to the pack as it became less saturated.

We used them primarily for sports injuries (sprained ankles, bruised hips, knee inflammation), but they also came in handy for digestive distress after too much sometimes food!

REST STOP

It's time for parents to take a break and digest information! Take 10 minutes of calm to Rest with the following questions:

1. **Assess the Inflammatory Potential of Current Habits**: Consider your child's diet, sleep, and activity levels. Are there certain foods or lifestyle habits (e.g., high sugar intake, sedentary behavior, stress) that may contribute to higher levels of inflammation? Reflect on which could be adjusted to promote a more anti-inflammatory environment.

2. **Reflect on Stress and Inflammation**: Stress is a significant contributor to inflammation. How do you and your child typically handle stress? Are there opportunities to introduce calming practices, like mindfulness or yoga, that could help reduce stress and, in turn, lower inflammation in your child's body?

Next, Stop for 10 minutes of quiet (sitting or slowly walking). Keep your mind as clear and open as possible, and just listen. Jot down or tell Siri to "make a note" of any responses that may arise. Because you've taken time to ponder calmly and quietly, these responses will most likely be less off-the-cuff and from a deeper level. They can give you clues as to the reasons behind your answers! Those clues, in turn, will reveal potential problematic thinking and can provide great direction on moving forward with the recommendations in this Step that would be the easiest to implement or fit best for your family!

ROADWORK

Inflammation Tracker Chart

Materials:

- Large sheet of paper or whiteboard

- Colorful markers or stickers.

Directions:

- **Create Sections:** Divide the chart into columns for each day of the week.

- **List Activities and Foods:** In the rows, list different activities, foods, and stress levels.

- **Track Symptoms:** Note any symptoms of inflammation (e.g., joint pain, irritability, digestive issues).

- **Identify Patterns:** At the end of the week, review the chart to identify any patterns or triggers.

This simple activity helps you keep track of your child's inflammation triggers and management techniques, making it easier to spot patterns and identify what works best for them.

SOUVENIR

You guessed it. Our suggested souvenir for the Inflammation Step is to get a castor oil pack for your household. Make one per the Roadwork section, or follow Alicia's suggestion and purchase one online: https://www.shopqueenofthethrones.com/. Either way, have your family begin to use castor oil packs and reap the many benefits regularly.

Next, we'll explore the intriguing world of body repair, focusing on strategies that promote healing and long-term health.

Chapter 10

Core Step Seven - Repair

"The DNA molecule is a work in progress, endlessly replicating, mutating, and evolving."

- James Watson, author of The Double Helix: A Personal Account of the Discovery of the Structure of DNA

SUMMARY - Travel Size Version

It's a post-school afternoon. Your 7-year-old son wants access to their digital device even though the household rule is "no screens on weekdays." You've consistently followed your guidelines, kept calm, expressed empathy, and offered other options. Nothing is helping, and the opposition is escalating to the point you've moved your toddler to the playpen to avoid an accidental collision with your careening-around-the-room-son. As you try to stay patient—despite your fatigue and weariness at the seemingly constant battle over screen time—you wonder if you can do more to help him manage these over-the-top moments.

The good news? Your child's body has an incredible ability to repair itself, particularly regarding their DNA, a factor that can impact behavior. In this Step, we explore DNA repair's crucial role in managing ADHD and how you can support this natural process.

Honoring Neurodiversity

First, you might wonder how DNA repair fits into a book focused on honoring neurodiversity, especially within an ADHD diagnosis. Our goal is truly to highlight the strengths and hidden potential often overlooked in ADHD discussions. We want our children with ADHD to see their value and believe in their strengths precisely as they are.

At the same time, we recognize that some aspects of ADHD, like impulsivity or overthinking, can be mismatched with particular environments, such as a traditional school setting or a team sport. Providing tools that optimize neurological functioning can help reduce stress and create a better fit between a child's needs and their environment.

Repair Genes

Remember the last time you needed to fix a torn screen door or patch an inflatable toy? Like you'd use a repair kit to mend that door or toy, your child's body has tools to repair DNA. Particular proteins find and fix DNA mistakes, keeping instructions clear. When repair genes work well, they improve attention, focus, and overall brain function.

Oxidative Stress

We'll explain oxidative stress and give you practical ways to minimize it, ensuring your child's brain stays in optimal condition.

Supplements that Support DNA Repair

We'll cover the body's built-in mechanisms for keeping things running smoothly and explore supplements that support DNA repair, offering simple ways to enhance your child's health.

DNA Detective

For our Roadwork activity, you and your child can become detectives, putting on your magnifying glasses and Sherlock Holmes hats for a fun, investigative exercise!

INFORMATION CENTER

Let's start by introducing you to Zach. He is a bright and energetic eight-year-old who's been struggling with ADHD. Zach's parents noticed he was having trouble focusing in school and was often restless at night. They decided to look into ways to support his DNA repair, hoping it might help with his symptoms. They began by including more colorful fruits and vegetables in his diet, aiming for at least five colors daily. Adding the extra produce wasn't just about making his plate look pretty; each of those different colored fruits and vegetables is packed with an array of antioxidants that help, in various ways, to neutralize oxidative stress.

Zach's folks also started limiting his screen time, especially before bed and encouraged outdoor activities like walking the nature trails in their neighborhood. Zach loved exploring the local park, and his parents noticed he seemed calmer and more focused afterward. They also consulted with a healthcare provider about adding supplements like astaxanthin and resveratrol to his routine. Over time, they saw significant improvements in Zach's behavior and overall well-being.

DNA repair might sound like something from an indie science fiction movie, but it's a natural and vital daily process in your child's (and every other) body. As a reminder, think of our DNA as the instruction manual for building and maintaining a human being. Over time, and due to factors like oxidative stress and environmental toxins, this manual can get damaged. Fortunately, our bodies have built-in repair mechanisms to fix these damages, ensuring everything runs smoothly.

First, let's look at some key genes involved in DNA repair and their impact on ADHD. One such gene is **SIRT6** (Sirtulin 6). SIRT6 is a multifunctional protein that plays a significant role in brain function, neurodevelopment, and neuroprotection. It also regulates stress responses and neuroinflammation, which, as we have seen before, are linked to ADHD. Think of SIRT6 as having a role in controlling inflammation and oxidative stress.

SIRT6 is a key gene involved in efficient DNA repair, as it recruits enzymes necessary for the repair process. When homozygous for the variant, this gene can increase oxidative stress, reduce DNA repair efficiency, and decrease autophagy—the body's "recycle and reuse" system. Reduced autophagy means cells discard components instead of recycling them, accumulating cellular waste that must be managed.

SIRT6 acts as a guardian of the genome, ensuring damage is addressed promptly. Efficient DNA repair is especially important in ADHD, as it supports the maintenance of proper brain function.

FOXO3 is an important gene associated with longevity and resistance to oxidative stress, the body's response to free radicals (more on this below). FOXO3 acts like the body's internal firefighter, responding to oxidative stress and assisting in DNA repair. Variations in this gene can significantly impact how effectively your child's body manages oxidative stress. In the case of a FOXO3 SNP, the normal coding (homozygous for normal) can be problematic, potentially leading to decreased DNA repair capacity, increased oxidative stress, and inflammation.

Then there's **BDNF** (Brain-Derived Neurotrophic Factor), a gene that plays a pivotal role in brain function and plasticity. BDNF is involved in the growth, maintenance, and survival of neurons, and it also plays a role in synaptic plasticity, which is essential for learning and memory. Think about BDNF as "miracle growth for the brain." In children with ADHD, optimal BDNF function is crucial for maintaining brain health and ensuring that neural connections are strong and adaptable. Variations in the BDNF gene can impact cognitive function and have been linked to ADHD symptoms.

SNP Peek - DNA Repair Genes

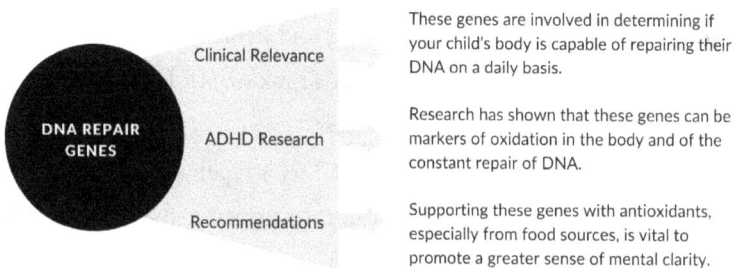

DNA REPAIR GENES

Clinical Relevance

These genes are involved in determining if your child's body is capable of repairing their DNA on a daily basis.

ADHD Research

Research has shown that these genes can be markers of oxidation in the body and of the constant repair of DNA.

Recommendations

Supporting these genes with antioxidants, especially from food sources, is vital to promote a greater sense of mental clarity.

Oxidation

Think of oxidation as the rust that forms on a bicycle left out in the rain or the browning that happens to an apple slice when exposed to the air. It's a natural process that occurs when your body uses oxygen to produce energy. This process generates reactive oxygen species (ROS), also known as free radicals, unstable molecules that can damage cells and DNA if not correctly managed. If this system is out of balance, it can impact DNA repair by causing breaks and mutations in the DNA strands, potentially leading to issues like cognitive decline and neurodevelopmental disorders, including ADHD.

Your body relies on antioxidants—compounds that neutralize ROS and protect cells from damage—to combat oxidative damage. Antioxidants are like the body's cleanup crew, swooping in to clear out harmful substances and keep everything running smoothly. This will date us, but think of that old Pac-Man video game as a visual of how antioxidants work!

Maintaining a high level of antioxidants is particularly important for children with ADHD, as oxidative stress can exacerbate symptoms and has been linked to ADHD. Foods rich in antioxidants, such as red and purple fruit—berries in particular—vegetables, nuts, and seeds, can help support this process.

Consider a colorful plate—we suggest aiming for the colors of the rainbow—as a toolbox full of different tools, each helping repair and maintain the body's intricate systems.

Beyond diet, other lifestyle factors can also support DNA repair. Reducing digital device use is one such factor. Excessive screen time can increase oxidative stress and disrupt sleep patterns, negatively impacting DNA repair. Encourage your child to take regular breaks from screens and avoid them before bedtime to help reduce these effects.

Another powerful tool is shinrin-yoku (i.e., forest bathing), which involves immersing oneself in nature and engaging all the senses. Forest bathing has been shown to reduce stress, lower blood pressure, and boost immune function, all of which can support DNA repair and overall well-being.

Finally, let's not forget the importance of quality sleep in DNA repair. Sleep is like a nightly reset button for your body, allowing it to repair and regenerate. During deep sleep, your body produces growth hormones that aid cell and tissue repair, including DNA repair. Ensuring that your child gets enough restful sleep is essential for maintaining their overall health and supporting their body's natural repair processes. (See Step Four - Sleep.)

Supplements to Support DNA Repair

Supplements can also support DNA repair. Astaxanthin, a powerful antioxidant found in certain algae, has been shown to protect cells from oxidative damage and support overall health. Resveratrol, another potent antioxidant mentioned in Step Six – Inflammation, is found in grapes and berries and can also support DNA repair, especially the BDNF gene.

Provided your child needs them, particularly if they have higher levels of oxidative stress, these supplements can be a valuable addition to a balanced diet.

TRAVELER ASSISTANCE

For this Step, we'll give you a simple, cost-effective method of cleaning your fruits and vegetables so you can maximize the antioxidant benefits of your produce.

Cleaning Produce with White Vinegar and Hydrogen Peroxide

A Virginia Tech study showed that separately spraying white vinegar and hydrogen peroxide is an effective way to clean produce and reduce harmful bacteria.

What You'll Need:

- White vinegar (undiluted)

- 3% hydrogen peroxide (undiluted, commonly found in drugstores)

- Two spray bottles

Instructions:

1. **Prepare the sprays:** Fill one spray bottle with undiluted white vinegar and the other with 3% hydrogen peroxide.

2. **Spray the produce:** Spray the produce thoroughly with the vinegar.

3. **Spray again:** Then immediately spray the produce with hydrogen peroxide.

4. **Rinse:** Let the sprays sit on the produce for a minute or two, then rinse

thoroughly under running water.

5. **Dry:** Pat the produce dry with a clean towel or paper towel.

This method is safe for most fruits and vegetables and more effective at reducing bacteria than using either solution alone or just water. However, it's important to note that the sprays should not be mixed in one bottle, as this can create an ineffective solution.

REST STOP

It's time for parents to take a break and digest information! Take 10 minutes of calm to Rest with the following questions:

1. **Reflect on the Importance of Rest and Recovery**: How much emphasis is placed on rest and recovery in your family's daily routine? Is there a balance between activity and downtime for yourself and your child? Or is what you are "doing" more highly valued than what you are "being?" Reflect on whether there might be opportunities to prioritize rest to allow the body and mind to repair more effectively.

2. **Consider Nutritional Support for Cellular Repair**: Think about the foods and nutrients most available in your household. Are there gaps in the diet that could affect your child's ability to repair tissues and cells (e.g., lack of protein, healthy fats, vitamins)? Reflect on small changes you could make to enhance your child's nutritional intake to support repair.

Next, Stop for 10 minutes of quiet (sitting or slowly walking). Keep your mind as clear and open as possible, and just listen. Jot down or tell Siri to "make a note" of any responses that may arise. Because you've taken time to ponder calmly and quietly, these responses will most likely be less off-the-cuff and from a deeper level. They can give you clues as to the reasons behind your answers! Those clues, in turn, will reveal potential problematic thinking and can provide great direction on moving forward with the recommendations in this Step that would be the easiest to implement or fit best for your family!

ROADWORK

Let's get hands-on with this Step's interactive activity, the DNA Repair Detective. Grab a notebook or a digital device, the magnifying glasses, and the detective hats we mentioned, and let's get started.

DNA Repair Detective

Materials:

Notebook or digital device, pen

Directions:

1. **Colorful Plate Challenge:** Each day, try to include at least five different colors of fruits and vegetables in your child's meals. Write down the colors and types of foods they eat.

2. **Screen-Free Hour:** Designate one hour before bedtime as screen-free time. Spend this hour doing calming activities like reading, drawing, or discussing the day.

3. **Outdoor Explorer:** Plan at least one weekly park or nature reserve trip. During the visit, encourage your child to use all their senses—listen to the birds, feel the bark on the trees, and smell the fresh air.

4. **Sleep Tracker:** Record your child's bedtime and wake-up time. Note any patterns or changes in their behavior after a good night's sleep.

5. **Supplement Check:** Consult your healthcare provider about adding antioxidants like astaxanthin and resveratrol to your child's diet. Note any changes in their behavior or overall health.

This activity helps you and your child become detectives, looking for clues about what best supports their DNA repair and overall health. It turns a complex process into a fun and engaging experience.

SOUVENIR

This Step's Souvenir is a simple yet powerful visualization exercise for your child that can help reinforce the connection between nourishing your body and supporting DNA repair. Depending on your child's age, adjust the visualization prompts so they can easily understand what to imagine.

Visualization Exercise: Supporting Your DNA Repair Through Nutrition

Don't underestimate the power of intention—visualizing the healing process can positively impact your mindset and overall well-being.

Step 1: Set the Stage for Relaxation

- Find a quiet, comfortable place for you and your child where you won't be disturbed for a few minutes. Sit or lie down in a relaxed position. You can close your eyes or keep them softly focused on a single point.

- Take a few deep, slow breaths. Inhale through your nose for a count of four, hold for a count of four, and then exhale slowly through your mouth. Repeat this until you feel calm and centered.

Step 2: Focus on Nourishing Your Body

- Consider the nutritious foods you've eaten recently or plan to eat—fruits, vegetables, proteins, healthy fats, and whole grains. Imagine how each food contains powerful nutrients—vitamins, minerals, antioxidants—your body craves for repair and growth.

- Picture these nutrients traveling through your bloodstream, heading to the areas of your body where they are most needed.

Step 3: Visualize DNA Repair

- Now, shift your focus to your DNA. Imagine your cells—millions of tiny units working around the clock to keep you healthy. Picture the DNA strands in each cell like blueprints that guide your body's functioning.

- Visualize any damaged DNA—think of it like a frayed shoelace in the blueprint. Now, imagine the nutrients from your food—vitamins like B12 and C, antioxidants like glutathione, and minerals like zinc—rushing in like tiny repair crews.

- See these nutrients repairing the DNA, mending the frayed parts, and making the strands strong and whole again. Picture them patching up any weak spots and restoring the DNA to its perfect state. Feel the sense of renewal and vitality as your cells regain their strength.

Step 4: Reinforce the Power of Food as Medicine

- Think about the words of Hippocrates: "Let thy food be thy medicine." Reflect on how nutritious foods are your body's tools for healing and repair. Each meal you eat is an opportunity to support your body's natural repair processes.

- Picture each bite of food you take in the future as another way to nourish your cells and enhance DNA repair. Imagine how these foods will continue to help your body grow stronger, healthier, and more resilient.

Step 5: Finish with Gratitude

- Take a moment to feel grateful for the food you have access to and for your body's incredible ability to heal and repair itself. When you're ready, take a few deep breaths and slowly open your eyes.

- As you and your child go about your day, carry this visualization with you, knowing that your food choices support your body at the cellular level.

We've now covered our introduction, Primer on ADHD Basics, and seven Core ELEVATE Steps. We'll wrap the book up with three short but important Supplemental Essentials: Behavioral and Educational Strategies, ADHD Family Dynamics, and Medical and Alternative Treatments. First up, Behavioral and Educational Strategies.

Chapter 11

Supplemental Essentials One - Behavioral and Educational Strategies

"For parents navigating the challenges of raising a child with ADHD, understanding the basics is crucial. Here are three key strategies that worked for me: 1) Build a strong foundation with structured routines and clear expectations to help your child manage daily tasks, 2) Reinforce positive behavior consistently to encourage self-regulation, and 3) Learn to recognize and address environmental triggers that can lead to hyperactivity or meltdowns."

                   - A parent in an ADHD group. Used with permission.

SUMMARY - Travel Size Version

While we have touched on behavior and educational strategies throughout the book because they are crucial for a child with ADHD, we will dedicate this whole chapter to addressing these essential keys. We will remind readers of strategies we've already covered and introduce several more.

Positive Behavioral Interventions for ADHD

Here, we'll provide suggestions for enhancing focus, reducing impulsivity, and managing intrusive thoughts and overthinking. Scroll through the options, chat with your child, and see which ones might fit.

Collaborating with Schools: Advocacy and IEPs

Understanding Individual Education Plans (IEPs) is crucial. These plans outline specific goals and accommodations to support your child's learning. We'll suggest ways to build collaborative relationships with educators and ensure everyone understands your child's needs.

Homework Strategies That Work for ADHD

Establishing a structured homework routine can make a world of difference. Stay tuned for strategies that help turn homework from a dreaded task into a manageable and, dare we say, enjoyable part of the day.

The Role of Technology in ADHD Education

Technology has both pros and cons for children with ADHD. While it offers tools for organization and learning, it can also be distracting. We'll help you balance technology's benefits and drawbacks, ensuring it remains a helpful tool.

Social Skills Training: Helping Your Child Navigate Friendships

Your child needs to develop healthy social skills to build relationships and self-esteem. This section provides strategies for helping your child develop and maintain friendships, boosting their confidence and social competence.

The Physiological Sigh, OCC Formula, and RESPOND Framework

Finally, we'll wrap up this chapter by introducing you to one of our favorite and most recommended breathing patterns, the Physiological Sigh, and an emotional exploration and regulation tool we have created, the RESPOND Framework.

INFORMATION CENTER

Positive Behavioral Interventions for ADHD

Before starting this section, we suggest you re-read the letter to parents in our Primer (p. 14). Why is that, you say? Well ...

We will be giving lots of suggestions, not all of which will work in your family situation and some of which you may have tried repeatedly or sporadically with little to no success thus far. This book, in general, and this chapter are meant to provide nonjudgmental and compassionate support for you and your child and to encourage you that our version of James Clear's Atomic Habits, "path of least resistance," is doing small, simple, sensible and sustainable tasks, over and over again. Re-reading that note to parents will remind you that this is not about perfection but progress and giving yourself lots of grace and kindness.

OK. Ready?

Your child—let's call him Josh—is having a meltdown because his reading assignment feels overwhelming. As your frustration rises, you take a deep breath and remember the power of positive behavioral interventions. These approaches aren't about punishment; they focus on reinforcing positive behaviors and responding thoughtfully to challenges. Think of yourself as a coach, guiding your child with empathy and understanding.

While reacting may mean yelling, retreating, or blaming, responding involves assessing the situation and choosing a constructive approach. Instead of losing patience, you could say, "I see you're frustrated. Let's work on this together." You can do breathing to calm yourself. Patterning the behavior you'd like your child to adopt can be helpful. Ensuring breakable items are out of reach makes sense. Turning on dance tunes and modeling the completion of a stress cycle with movement (more on that in the ADHD Family Dynamics chapter's Souvenir) could be beneficial. Any of these shifts in your behavior could make a significant difference in your child's behavior.

When dopamine levels are low, your child might instinctively seek quick fixes to boost dopamine, such as playing video games, consuming sugary snacks, or engaging in challenging behaviors like arguing, name-calling, or physical confrontation. These behaviors serve as short-term solutions to satisfy their brain's craving for dopamine but can have long-term negative consequences.

Understanding this dynamic allows you to create an environment that supports healthier ways to increase dopamine. Encourage physical exercise, engaging hobbies, creative play, or even a quick rope-skipping session, which can naturally enhance dopamine levels while promoting emotional regulation and positive behaviors.

Many parents of children with ADHD have found that implementing a reward system can be transformative. Immediate rewards like a sticker or extra play-time offer quick motivation, while delayed rewards like weekend outings build anticipation. Quality time with your child is a highly recommended reward, as endorsed by Drs. Gordon Neufeld and Gabor Maté in their book *Hold Onto Your Kids: Why Parents Need to Matter More Than Peers* (one of my [Brenda's] favorite and most recommended parenting books ever!). Here are five ways to do this:

1. Schedule a weekly game night.

2. Plan a monthly park outing.

3. Set aside 15 minutes of undivided attention daily.

4. Cook a meal together.

5. Create art projects side by side.

These moments strengthen your bond while rewarding positive behavior.

Behavioral modification techniques, like token economies or contingency contracts, can be adapted for home and school. A token economy lets your child earn points for tasks, which can be exchanged for rewards. Response cost systems involve losing privileges for negative behavior, and contingency contracts outline expectations and rewards. Monitor progress by setting clear goals and tweaking systems when necessary to keep things effective and engaging.

Techniques for Enhancing Focus, Reducing Impulsivity, and Managing Intrusive Thoughts

As previously mentioned, Cognitive Behavioral Techniques (CBT) are excellent tools for improving focus and reducing impulsivity. Think of CBT as helping your child become a "detective" who uncovers behavior triggers and develops management strategies. Self-monitoring can be simple, like using a chart to track completed tasks or problem-solving challenges like forgetting homework. Make it engaging by brainstorming solutions and role-playing outcomes.

CBT can also be used to address overthinking and intrusive thoughts. A Thought-Emotion Chart helps younger children map out their thoughts and feelings, making it easier for them to manage their emotions. For example, writing down "I'm scared of starting swimming lessons" and identifying the associated emotion helps create awareness of thought patterns.

Use the mindfulness techniques previously discussed, too. They help children stay present and reduce mental clutter. Mindful breathing involves slow, deep breaths, focusing on the sensation of air entering and leaving the body. Guided imagery takes your child on a mental journey, like imagining a peaceful beach, while body scans build awareness of physical sensations and promote relaxation.

Modifying your child's environment can enhance focus. Organize spaces with bins and shelves to minimize distractions, and use noise-canceling headphones during homework time. Establishing a consistent routine—like having a set sleep hygiene routine and regular bedtime—creates a structure that reduces anxiety. Planning the day together and clearly stating expectations helps children feel secure and prepared.

Timers and alarms are great tools to manage tasks. Use a timer for focused homework periods, followed by short breaks. Musical alarms can signal transitions between activities, helping your child adjust smoothly. For example, set an alarm five minutes before the end of playtime to ease into required reading time.

Breathwork can help manage intrusive thoughts and overthinking. Patterns like the "4-7-8" method (inhale for four seconds, hold for seven, exhale for eight) can calm the nervous system. "Bunny Breaths" (three quick sniffs through the nose and one long exhale) and "Square Breathing" (inhale for four seconds, hold for four, exhale for four, hold for four) are fun, effective techniques.

We mentioned Non-Sleep Deep Rest (NSDR) in Step Five – Calm, but here, we want to emphasize its ability to help your child manage overthinking. NSDR mimics some of the benefits of sleep by slowing brain wave frequency and fostering relaxation and mental clarity. Guided NSDR sessions, often available on platforms like YouTube, typically begin with a soothing voice, leading participants into a profoundly restful state. This is followed by a focus on different body parts or sensations, promoting mindfulness and grounding. This practice helps your child relax quickly and deeply and improves focus, memory, and overall cognitive function.

Mindfulness-Based Cognitive Strategies combine mindfulness with cognitive techniques. "Thought Labeling" helps children identify their thoughts (e.g., "I'm having a worried thought"), giving them distance from these thoughts. "Anchoring" focuses attention on a physical sensation (e.g., feet on the ground), bringing awareness back to the present.

The Emotional Freedom Technique (EFT), or "tapping," involves tapping specific body points while focusing on an emotion or issue. This technique can help manage intrusive thoughts by reducing their emotional intensity.

Techniques for Enhancing Focus, Reducing Impulsivity, and Managing Intrusive Thoughts

Cognitive Behavioral Techniques - CBT

Mindfulness

Modifying the Environment

Timers and Alarms

Breathwork

Non-Sleep Deep Rest

Meditation

Emotional Freedom Technique

Collaborating with Schools: Advocacy and IEPs

When your child is diagnosed with ADHD, it's natural to feel a mix of emotions—from relief to concern about potential labeling and stigma. These feelings are understandable, and exploring them with curiosity can help you advocate more effectively on their behalf. Writing or discussing your thoughts with a friend or counselor can bring clarity, some measure of peace, and a concrete action plan.

Individualized Education Plans (IEPs), crucial for many children with ADHD, may be a part of your action plan. These documents outline specific goals, accommodations, and strategies to meet each child's unique educational needs.

While the plan's name or terminology may vary across countries (or even across states or provinces), the core idea remains: to create a supportive environment tailored to your child's learning style. When this book was published, IEPs were legally mandated in the U.S. to ensure students received the necessary resources to succeed.

Effective advocacy requires preparation and persistence. Gather relevant documents, such as diagnoses and previous assessments, and communicate clearly and concisely with school staff. A checklist can help organize key discussion points and desired accommodations.

Knowing the types of practices and routines that can help calm your child (e.g., manipulating a stress ball, chewing on a fabric necklace), allowing their energy to be safely dispensed (e.g., a 5-minute run around the playground, a minute of skipping in the coat room), and offering suggestions for the plan can be helpful if it is a match for the way your child functions best.

Building a collaborative relationship with educators is vital. Approach meetings with a partnership mindset, emphasizing the shared goal of supporting your child. Regular communication through emails, phone calls, or meetings helps keep everyone on the same page.

Collaboration, however, goes beyond the initial IEP meeting—it's about creating an ongoing support network, including teachers, counselors, and special education staff. Regularly reviewing and adjusting the IEP ensures it stays aligned with your child's evolving needs. Be proactive in suggesting changes based on observations at home and request periodic updates to stay informed.

Homework Strategies That Work for ADHD

Establishing a structured homework routine can turn a daily struggle into a manageable task. Set a consistent homework time when your child is most alert and create a quiet, clutter-free space dedicated to work. This structure reduces the anxiety of unpredictability, making it easier for your child to focus. It also gives you a sense of control and organization in your efforts to help your child manage their homework.

Breaking tasks into smaller parts is crucial. Large assignments can be overwhelming and lead to many children's default modes, such as procrastination or avoidance. Teach your child to divide homework into smaller, manageable steps, like reading a chapter daily, outlining ideas, and writing one paragraph at a time. Use organizational charts or "sticky" notes to visually map out these tasks, providing a sense of accomplishment with each small step.

Visual aids are powerful tools for organization. Use charts, color-coded folders, and planners to track assignments. A whiteboard or calendar can visually outline tasks for the week, helping your child stay on track. Breaking assignments into daily goals provides a clear roadmap.

Use creativity to keep your child engaged. Incorporate frequent breaks to avoid burnout—set 20-minute work periods followed by five-minute movement breaks. If your child feels stuck on a task, switch activities and return to it later. Integrating physical movement—like hopping on one foot while reciting spelling words—or regular small rewards—placing an almond or raisin at the end of each line of printing practice to be eaten when the line is completed—makes homework more interactive and less tedious, inspiring you to think outside the box and making learning fun and engaging for your child.

The Role of Technology in ADHD Education

Technology can be both a help and a hindrance for children with ADHD. Digital tools like tablets and smart boards can assist with organization and make tasks more engaging, and many apps are available that can help a child focus. Technology can also improve communication between parents, students, and educators.

That said, because of some of the negative impacts of screen use on children, in general, but in particular in children with ADHD, we recommend minimal use of digital devices with your child.

One primary reason is that even educational video games, social media use, and other forms of technology can lead to distraction or become a constant go-to mini-dopamine hit.

One of technology's prime attractions for people is that it provides fast, frequent rewards, stimulating dopamine in the brain's reward pathways. For children with ADHD, who may have lower baseline dopamine levels or dopamine dysregulation, this constant stimulation can become especially appealing (AKA tantrums when you try to call an end to screen use!).

Over time, the brain can start to "wire in" this need for frequent dopamine boosts, making it harder for the child to tolerate less immediately rewarding activities, such as homework, chores, or a family walk. This reliance on quick dopamine sources can also lower overall motivation for tasks that don't offer the same kind of instant gratification, potentially deepening symptoms of inattention, impulsivity, and difficulty focusing.

If you end up using screen time with your child (which, as mentioned in Step Three – Sleep, can sometimes be supportive), set boundaries to ensure technology remains a helpful tool and not a source of distraction or constant dopamine release.

Social Skills Training: Helping Your Child Navigate Friendships

Because some ADHD behaviors can be a mismatch in social interactions, they can lead to misunderstandings or isolation. Social skills training can help children navigate these challenges and form meaningful connections.

Check online for programs that cover skills like starting conversations, taking turns, recognizing social cues, and resolving conflicts, or use a low-tech practice that I (Brenda) used with one of our sons, who was very shy as a youngster. As he often hesitated to speak up or participate in conversations with new people, we practiced good communication skills with a tennis ball game. My husband or I would begin with the tennis ball in our hand, start a conversation, and then toss the ball to our son. He would need to respond with a statement, question, or follow-up comment to the initial statement and then throw the ball back to us. By tossing the ball back and forth to move the conversation forward, our son was able to feel more comfortable with his communication skills while having fun and a positive 1-1 parenting time.

Games like "Tennis Ball Talk," role-playing, and family discussion times allow children to practice and internalize these skills in a safe, supportive environment.

Role-playing scenarios are especially effective for practicing social interactions. You can simulate situations like introducing themselves to a new friend, resolving a disagreement, or asking to join a group activity. Practicing these responses in controlled environments helps your child apply them in real life, building confidence.

Facilitating positive peer interactions is vital. Supervised playdates offer a safe space for children to practice social skills with peers. Cooperative activities like building a fort or playing a board game encourage teamwork and positive interaction. Peer buddy systems, group activities, or sports teams help your child connect with others in structured, supportive settings, fostering their social competence and confidence.

TRAVELER ASSISTANCE
The Physiological Sigh: A Simple, Powerful Tool for Instant Calm

The Physiological Sigh is one of our favorite breathing patterns. It is a natural, automatic reflex that your body uses to regulate stress and calm the nervous system. You or your child may have noticed it when you're feeling deeply emotional or right before you fall asleep—it's that spontaneous, long exhale after taking a deep breath.

Science shows that this reflex can be a powerful tool for reducing stress, calming anxiety, and improving focus. Let's examine how it works and how you and your child can intentionally use it to bring calm into your daily lives.

Background: How the Physiological Sigh Works

Your lungs comprise millions of tiny air sacs called alveoli, which expand when you breathe in and collapse when you breathe out. Sometimes, when we're stressed, anxious, or even just sitting for long periods, these tiny sacs don't fully release carbon dioxide, which builds up in the body and can cause feelings of tension or stress.

The Physiological Sigh works by taking a deep, intentional double inhale (one long inhale followed by a quick second inhale) and then a slow, controlled exhale. This double breath helps fully inflate the alveoli and release excess carbon dioxide, resetting your body's oxygen levels and calming the nervous system. The result? Almost immediate relaxation and focus.

Why It's Effective
- **Restores balance:** The double inhale followed by a long exhale helps release trapped air from the lungs, bringing in more oxygen and balanc-

ing carbon dioxide levels.

- **Activates the parasympathetic nervous system:** This is the "rest, digest, feed, and breed" part of the autonomic nervous system. It helps calm the heart rate and reduce stress.

- **Instant relief:** After one or two physiological sighs, you'll feel more relaxed. It's quick, easy, and can be done anytime, anywhere.

How to Perform the Physiological Sigh

1. **Find a comfortable position:** You can do this sitting, standing, or lying down. Relax your body and drop your shoulders away from your ears.

2. **First inhale:** Take a long, deep breath through your nose, filling your lungs almost to total capacity.

3. **Second inhale:** Take a quick inhale without exhaling to inflate your lungs fully. This extra breath should feel like a "top-up" of air.

4. **Exhale slowly:** Now, exhale all the air slowly and steadily through your mouth. Make the exhale longer than your inhale. Let it all out.

5. **Repeat as needed:** Repeat this process 1-3 times, or more, until you feel calm and relaxed.

When to Use the Physiological Sigh

You or your child can use the Physiological Sigh anytime you feel stressed, anxious, or overwhelmed or need a quick reset to refocus. It's particularly beneficial:

- Before bed to help wind down and prepare for sleep

- During moments of frustration, tension, or anxiety

- Before a test, meeting, or performance to calm your nerves

- When transitioning between tasks to clear the mind and reset

Once your child masters the Sigh, they can use this virtually unde-tectable-to-others calming technique in the classroom, on the playground, or in any situation that calls for focus or a reset of emotions.

REST STOP

It's time for parents to take a break and digest information! Take 10 minutes of calm to Rest with the following questions:

1. **Reflect on your own childhood experiences with discipline:** How did your caregivers approach behavioral challenges when you were growing up? Are there any patterns from your past that you've car-ried into your parenting style, especially when dealing with your child's ADHD-related behaviors? Are those patterns a fit or a mismatch with your child's way of seeing and experiencing the world?

2. **Examine your expectations:** Are your current expectations of your child's behavior aligned with their developmental stage and how their ADHD impacts them? Could adjusting these expectations foster more patience and positivity in your interactions?

Next, Stop for 10 minutes of quiet (sitting or slowly walking). Keep your mind as clear and open as possible, and just listen. Jot down or tell Siri to "make a note" of any responses that may arise. Because you've taken time to ponder calmly and quietly, these responses will most likely be less off-the-cuff and from a deeper level. They can give you clues as to the reasons behind your answers! Those clues, in turn, will reveal potential problematic thinking and can provide great direction on moving forward with the recommendations in this chapter that would be the easiest to implement or fit best for your family!

ROADWORK

Emotions and Achievements Chart

Materials:

- Large sheet of paper or whiteboard

- Colorful markers or stickers

Directions:

- **Create Sections:** Divide the chart into two columns—one for emotions and one for achievements.

- **Track Emotions:** Have your child write down or draw how they feel each day (happy, frustrated, calm).

- **List Achievements:** Have your child note any successes, no matter how small.

- **Celebrate Together:** Use stickers or drawings to celebrate achievements and discuss emotions.

SOUVENIR

One of the emotional exploration and regulation tools I (Brenda) have often used with clients and group participants is a concept I created called the OCC Formula: Observations, Curiosity, and Compassion. It is a simple three-step action plan that allows you to be gracious and compassionate with yourself as you sort through more challenging moments.

However, for parenting children with ADHD, we have expanded the formula to include aspects of Effective Parenting and work by Dr. Ross W. Greene (author of *The Explosive Child*) and created a simple seven-step framework. Our RESPOND framework focuses on emergency emotional dysregulation moments (e.g., meltdowns). This approach is designed to help parents respond to their child's challenging behavior with understanding and structure while being flexible enough to adapt to everyday parenting or parenting children who do not have ADHD.

The RESPOND Framework

(Reflect, Empathize, Support, Plan, Organize, Navigate, Debrief)

1. REFLECT: Pause Before Reacting

Before responding to your child's meltdown, take a moment to assess your own emotional state. Remember, your emotional well-being is crucial to this process.

What to do:

- Ensure the situation is safe (e.g., remove breakable objects or potentially damaging projectiles, move a younger sibling to their playpen or crib so they are out of harm's way)

- Take a deep breath or count to 10.

- Remind yourself that your child's behavior is communication, not defiance.

Why it works: Pausing prevents escalation and allows you to approach the situation objectively.

2. EMPATHIZE: Acknowledge the Emotion

Identify and validate your child's emotions, even if their reaction seems disproportionate.

What to say:

- "I can see you're feeling really upset right now."

- "It's hard when things don't go how we want them to."

Why it works: This helps diffuse tension and lets your child feel seen and understood. Your empathy is a powerful tool that builds a connection essential for moving forward.

3. SUPPORT: Provide a Calming Tool or Strategy

Help your child regulate their emotions by offering a tangible way to calm down.

What to do:

- Offer choices: "Do you want to sit in your calm corner or do a Physiological Sigh together?"

- Use sensory tools like a weighted blanket, stress ball, or a simple breathing exercise.

Why it works: Dysregulated kids can't process verbal instructions. Providing a tool or activity engages their body and mind, helping them transition from emotional overwhelm to calmness.

4. PLAN: Problem-Solve Together

Once your child has calmed down, collaborate on a plan to address the situation.

What to ask:

- "What was hard for you in that moment?"

- "What might have led up to it?"

- "What could we do next time to make it easier?"

Why it works: By involving your child, you teach problem-solving and give them control over their environment.

5. ORGANIZE: Adjust the Environment

Modify the physical or emotional environment to reduce overstimulation and set the stage for calm.

What to do:

- Declutter the space or dim harsh lighting.

- Provide sensory aids, like noise-canceling headphones or a quiet corner.

Why it works: A structured and calming environment helps regulate arousal levels, making it easier for your child to regain control and focus.

6. NAVIGATE: Guide Toward Resolution

Help your child transition back to their day and take steps toward resolving the situation.

What to do:

- Identify immediate actions to address any lingering issues (e.g., cleaning up a mess and repairing relationships).

- Reinforce positive actions they can take moving forward.

- Offer reassurance that they can handle challenges with your support.

Why it works: By guiding your child back to a sense of normalcy and responsibility, you instill confidence in their ability to recover from difficulties and move forward constructively.

7. DEBRIEF: Reflect and Learn Together

After the incident, take time to reflect on what happened and discuss how to handle similar situations in the future.

What to ask yourself and your child:

- "What worked well this time, and what could we improve?"

- "How can we approach this differently next time?"

- For yourself: "Did I remain calm and supportive, or are there moments I could improve?"

Why it works: Reflection fosters growth for both you and your child. Learning from the incident strengthens your ability to handle future challenges and helps your child develop emotional resilience and problem-solving skills.

Emergency Response Mnemonic: RESPOND

When your child is overwhelmed, remember to RESPOND:

- **Reflect** (pause and check yourself)

- **Empathize** (validate their feelings)

- **Support** (offer a calming tool or strategy)

- **Plan** (collaborate on next steps)

- **Organize** (adjust the environment for calm)

- **Navigate** (guide your child to a sense of normalcy and responsibility)

- **Debrief** (reflect together for future success)

The RESPOND method provides both a structured approach to handling meltdowns and a philosophy of parenting that fosters growth, connection, and resilience in children with ADHD ... and is a natural segue to our next Supplemental Essential, ADHD Family Dynamics.

Chapter 12

Supplemental Essentials Two - ADHD Family Dynamics

"Family is not an important thing; it's everything."
- Michael J. Fox, author of Lucky Man: A Memoir

S UMMARY - Travel Size Version

Managing family dynamics when you have a child with ADHD can be challenging. It seems you are constantly trying to explain ADHD behavior to other children in the family and have them express empathy for a sibling that has recently been verbally or even physically abusive to them. At the same time, in your child with ADHD's calmer moments, you try to help them understand why a sibling might be pulling back from play or interaction with them.

It's not an easy journey, but in this chapter, we'll try to break it down into manageable pieces.

Sibling Relationships: Balancing Attention and Addressing Resentment

Balancing attention between children can be difficult in families with a child with ADHD, and no one will get it right all the time (believe us ... we know!).

In this section, we'll give some tips on involving siblings in ADHD management strategies and providing them with emotional support to help reduce resentment and strengthen family bonds.

Strategies for Parental Self-Care and Emotional Health

Here, we will look at ways that parents of children with ADHD can prioritize self-care. We're also big fans of setting realistic parenting expectations and practicing self-compassion, as those skills are vital for managing the emotional challenges of raising a child with ADHD.

Family Activities That Support ADHD Management

In this section, we'll show how family meetings and educational activities can foster communication and create fun, supportive environments for the whole family.

Handling Conflicts: Tips for Peaceful Resolution

Teaching conflict resolution skills, such as active listening and calm problem-solving, can de-escalate tense situations. These skills can be used by the whole family. We will cover practices to foster a more peaceful household and stronger relationships.

Building a Supportive Home Environment and Communicating About ADHD with Extended Family and Friends

An ADHD-friendly home with organized spaces and routines helps children feel secure. We'll suggest ways to address sensory needs and use inclusive decision-making.

Because most people have both nuclear and extended family members, we'll also discuss educating extended family and friends about ADHD.

Empowering Your Child to Self-Advocate

We'll examine the value of self-advocacy in empowering children with ADHD to communicate their needs confidently.

Completing the Stress Cycle

This chapter's Roadwork outlines the essential concept of completing the stress cycle. We'll explain what that means and give you various ways to model and teach your child how to do so.

INFORMATION CENTER

You're in the middle of a family game night. The board game pieces are scattered, your youngest child is giggling uncontrollably, and your older child, who has ADHD, is on the verge of exploding because they didn't get the card they wanted. As you try to keep the peace, you can't help but notice your middle child sitting quietly in the corner, looking like they'd rather be anywhere else. Balancing attention and addressing confusion and resentment among siblings is a common challenge for families with a child with ADHD. Still, there are strategies to ensure everyone feels valued and loved.

Sibling Relationships: Balancing Attention and Addressing Resentment

Equitable attention is crucial in families with children with ADHD, and scheduled one-on-one time with each child can make a world of difference. That sentence seems so straightforward and innocuous. However, can we also interject here and say this can be challenging or even impossible some weeks?

In the early days of Rachel's Lyme disease intersection with her undiagnosed ADHD, the most challenging household situations revolved around figuring out the best treatment approach for the Lyme, sorting the way to fit those treatments into our budget, dealing with the severe physical and emotional symptoms she was experiencing, trying to help her deal with the uncertainties of her future with the disease, all the while trying to respond rather than react to her Lyme rages that were often directed at the two siblings still living at home. Though we knew spending time with Joel and Rebekah was crucial, some weeks, there simply weren't enough hours to fit everything in.

Even before Rachel's encounter with a tick, however, there were multiple apples (e.g., a new baby in the house, a child's weekend sports tournament, another child's speech challenges) that upset the balancing-attention-with-all-the-kids apple cart.

Therefore, note that we are saying one-on-one time with all your children is super important and that we have a lot of grace for the times when it doesn't happen.

Here are some tips to have them happen more often than not: consider designating specific days or times for individual activities that cater to each child's interests. It could be a Saturday morning brunch date with your youngest or a Wednesday evening soccer practice with your middle child. These moments strengthen your bond and reassure each child that they are special and cared for. Though the time allotments might not work out equitably each week, the overall goal is to create a level playing field where no child feels like they're always the second fiddle to their ADHD sibling.

Educating siblings about ADHD in an age-appropriate manner is also important and can foster understanding and empathy. Use the different vs. deficit model we've discussed and explain that ADHD is a difference in how the brain works, not a bad behavior. Use simple analogies, like how some people need hearing aids to hear better while others need help to focus and stay calm. These types of explanations help demystify ADHD and reduce the stigma. Encourage questions and open discussions, allowing siblings to express their feelings and frustrations. By providing them with the knowledge to understand their sibling's behavior, you help build a compassionate and supportive family environment.

Involving siblings in age-appropriate ADHD management strategies can also help. Suddenly, they are part of the solution, not sidelined bystanders. Include them in setting up routines, creating visual schedules, and even participating in counseling sessions if appropriate. This involvement can increase their sense of "place" and reduce feelings of alienation or resentment.

For instance, if your ADHD child has a specific calming technique that works for them—a physiological sigh, for example—have them teach it to their siblings so they can use it themselves or remind their sibling with ADHD to use it when a situation threatens to get out of hand. Having a shared set of tools in the family toolkit not only fosters teamwork but also strengthens sibling bonds, turning potential sources of conflict into opportunities for collaboration.

Support for siblings is just as important as support for a child with ADHD. Look into resources such as siblings of children with ADHD support groups or activities where they can express their feelings and experiences. These groups provide a safe space for siblings to share their frustrations, learn coping strategies, and realize they are not alone.

Activities like art therapy, sports, or a simple journaling routine can help them constructively process their emotions. Acknowledge their feelings of embarrassment, frustration, or guilt and reassure them that it's okay to feel this way.

Strategies for Parental Self-Care and Emotional Health

The harsh reality of parenting is that our children's behaviors often mirror ours. We make that statement without judgment or finger-pointing. As the saying goes, we have been there, done that.

Instead, the mirroring analogy simply exposes the responsibility we, as parents, have to behave as well as we possibly can with our current set of tools and to grow and learn best practices to become the healthiest version of ourselves—body, mind, and spirit.

To do that, we need to move the concept of "taking care of ourselves" from the category of "luxury" to that of "necessity."

When you prioritize self-care, whatever that looks like for you, you're better equipped to handle the ups and downs of parenting a child with ADHD. Managing stress and health impacts your ability to be present and supportive of your children. Think of it like the proverbial oxygen mask on an airplane—you must secure your mask before assisting others around you.

By taking time for yourself, you are not being selfish; you are ensuring that you have the strength and patience to be the best version of your parent-self.

Engaging in self-care activities doesn't need to be elaborate or time-consuming. Regular exercise, even a 10-minute brisk walk or exercise "snacks" like a set of 10 body-weight squats once every hour, can help clear your mind and boost your mood. When your child with ADHD needs an exercise break, have them hop on their bike and jog beside you for a few laps around the block.

Hobbies that you enjoy, such as gardening, knitting, or reading, provide a much-needed mental break and can be done while children play outside (gardening) or while they are at school or in bed (knitting, reading).

Building emotional support networks is another crucial aspect of self-care. Socializing with friends, even virtually, can offer emotional support and remind you that you're not alone. Joining groups in person or online can provide a sense of community and understanding. Counseling can help you deal with past traumas and grow in the depth and breadth of your self-regulation. These activities help maintain your emotional health, making you more resilient and patient when dealing with the daily challenges of parenting a child with ADHD.

Online communities dedicated to parents of children with ADHD can be invaluable for sharing experiences and advice (e.g., the many excellent Parenting Children with ADHD Facebook groups). These networks remind you that seeking help is okay and that you don't have to navigate this journey alone.

Setting realistic expectations for yourself and your parenting is also vital. It's easy to fall into the trap of self-blame or guilt when things don't go as planned, and they are often not going to go as planned! Understand that parenting a child with ADHD comes with its own set of challenges and unpredictabilities. Give yourself grace and remember that perfection isn't the goal.

Celebrate small victories and give yourself grace and compassion when things don't go as hoped. Setting achievable goals and being kind to yourself can reduce feelings of pressure and guilt, making the journey more manageable and allowing you to see the good, joyful, productive, and loving moments more easily.

One important final note on self-care: ADHD brains require more than typical self-awareness, self-care, and self-compassion when things don't go as planned. Caring for yourself is also modeling a critical skill for your child with ADHD.

Family Activities That Support ADHD Management

Choosing family activities that recognize your child with ADHD's strengths and interests can be very beneficial. Opt for inclusive activities where they can fully engage and thrive. If your child loves being outdoors, consider nature hikes or beach time. These activities provide sensory experiences and physical exercise, which benefit ADHD management. For more artistically inclined children, family art projects, jewelry-making classes, or dance lessons can harness that creative energy. The goal is to choose activities where your child with ADHD feels successful and included, boosting their confidence and reducing frustration while, at the same time, choosing an activity that also meets the needs and interests of your other children.

As we've discussed, it's crucial to balance structured activities with flexibility. Structure provides predictability, which is calming for children with ADHD. However, flexibility allows for adjustments based on their day-to-day moods and energy levels. Plan activities with clear start and end times, but be willing to adapt. For example, if a planned trip to the zoo seems overwhelming on a particular day, a quiet picnic in the park might be a better alternative.

Make good use of educational activities, too, as they can be informative and fun. Board games that involve strategy and teamwork can teach valuable skills while keeping the family engaged. It can take some work to find games that don't foster frustration in your child with ADHD, but keep trying various options until one or two lands.

Science experiments at home can turn learning into a hands-on adventure. Cooking or baking can improve math skills by measuring ingredients and following recipes. These activities support your child's learning and create memorable (and potentially tasty!) family moments.

Regular family meetings can also significantly affect family dynamics and emotional state. These meetings allow all family members to contribute to activity planning and discuss any needed adjustments. Start with a simple agenda: review the past week, discuss upcoming events, and address concerns. Use a visual schedule to keep everyone on track. Encourage each child to share their feelings and suggestions. This practice fosters open communication and ensures that everyone feels heard and valued.

Handling Conflicts: Tips for Peaceful Resolution

Conflict resolution skills are vital, especially in families with an ADHD member where a typical Saturday morning can include a simple disagreement about chores escalating into a full-blown kicking, screaming, toy-flinging argument.

Teaching effective conflict resolution starts with active listening. This means genuinely hearing what the other person is saying without interrupting or planning your subsequent reply. Encourage your family to use "I" statements like, "I feel upset when ..." to express feelings without blaming. Make sure everyone knows the house rules—they could, perhaps, be posted in clear view—along with the consequences for breaking them. When emotions run high, calm problem-solving can prevent conflicts from spiraling out of control. Teach your children to take a deep breath, step back, and think before reacting.

De-escalation techniques can be lifesavers during moments of high tension. For instance, having a predefined signal, like a hand gesture, a specific word, or Rachel and my (Brenda) "pinkie swear," can indicate the need for a break. When things get heated, taking a timeout lets everyone cool down and gather their thoughts.

Calming strategies like deep breathing exercises or soothing music can help shift the mood. Encourage your child to identify and use these techniques when they feel overwhelmed. This process empowers them to manage their emotions better and reduces the likelihood of conflicts escalating.

Mediation can significantly improve family dynamics by resolving ongoing conflicts. Family therapy or counseling provides a neutral space for everyone to express their feelings and resolve issues. A trained mediator can help guide the conversation, ensuring everyone feels heard and respected. Mediation can also teach valuable skills like empathy and compromise, which are essential for healthy relationships. By normalizing mediation, you create an environment where seeking help is seen as a strength, not a weakness.

At one point, Rachel and I (Brenda) worked together with a psychologist. Even all these years later, we agree that the time was well spent, as our communication improved, along with our understanding and empathy for each other.

We'd also encourage you to have your family view disagreements as an opportunity to better understand each other's perspectives and needs. After a conflict, hold a family meeting to discuss what happened and how it could be handled differently next time. This reflection fosters a mindset of continuous growth and helps build stronger relationships.

Conflicts are inevitable, but how your family handles them can make all the difference. Approaching disputes with an open mind and a willingness to learn can turn challenges into valuable life lessons for everyone involved.

Building a Supportive Home Environment

Creating an ADHD-friendly home setup can significantly impact your household's daily life. To follow are a few reminders we've touched on elsewhere in the book, this time outlined in "point of performance" terms, an organization principle referring to creating organizational systems that work directly where and when tasks need to happen.

Used in various contexts but highlighted for use with ADHD brains by authors like Susan C. Pinsky in her book *Organizing Solutions for People with ADHD*, point of performance is an approach that aligns with ADHD traits such as difficulty with working memory, executive functioning challenges and time blindness (difficulty in perceiving the passage of time, often leading to challenges in planning, prioritizing, or meeting deadlines), and can be an important and effective guiding principle for ADHD management.

Keep Tools and Supplies Where They are Needed:

- Designated areas for specific activities and ensure everything needed for tasks in that area are readily accessible, in that same area.

Use Visual Reminders:

- Start by organizing spaces with clear labels, color-code items, and create checklists. Visual systems are often key for ADHD brains to best function as they often don't do well with an "out of sight, out of mind" approach.

Simplify Systems:

- As one of our moms recounted earlier, if dirty socks keep being left all over the house, put a dirty sock basket by the shoe rack. And note, make it a basket, not a drawer, to make it easier to see and use.

Minimize Clutter:

- ADHD brains can be overwhelmed by too many options. To prevent this, Keep it Super Simple (i.e., the KISS principle), with clear surfaces and rarely used items stored away.

Create Zones:

- Organize the space by activity, with a homework zone, a meal-prep zone, and a quiet zone with bins containing calming activities such as books, puzzles, headphones for use with binaural beats, and weighted blankets.

Routine and structure are your best friends when it comes to managing ADHD. Establishing consistent daily routines provides stability and predictability that can be incredibly calming for your child. Simple things like having a set meal time, homework, free play, and bedtime can create a rhythm that makes the day more manageable. Use visual schedules to outline the day's activities, and involve your child in developing these plans, giving them a sense of ownership. Consistency is key; the more predictable the environment, the less room for anxiety and confusion.

Addressing sensory considerations is also crucial. As one mom mentioned, her son had a high sensitivity to fabrics and seams in his clothing (especially socks). Even if your child can't describe why they don't want to wear something, it could be a clue to sensory challenges.

Children with ADHD often have heightened sensitivities to their surroundings. Soft blues and greens can create a calming, soothing atmosphere. Rugs, curtains, and noise-canceling headphones help minimize noise and distractions. Providing sensory tools like fidget toys, stress balls, and weighted blankets can offer comfort and help your child self-regulate. Note that different organizations (e.g., therapyBC.ca) set guidelines for the maximum weight of a blanket per child's body weight and provide information on maximum time use.

Pay attention to lighting as well; natural light is best, but if that's not possible, opt for soft, warm lighting that mimics natural sunlight.

Inclusive decision-making can also help transform your household dynamics. Involve the entire family in decisions about home arrangements and rules, ensuring everyone's needs and opinions are considered. Hold family meetings where members can voice their thoughts and contribute to the discussion, actions that foster a sense of belonging and respect. For example, if you're reorganizing the family room, ask for input on the layout and choose a setup that works for everyone. Making decisions together strengthens family bonds and ensures the home environment supports everyone's well-being.

Communicating About ADHD with Extended Family and Friends

Navigating conversations about ADHD with extended family and friends can be challenging. You might find yourself explaining your child's behavior during a holiday family gathering or deflecting well-meaning but misguided advice from a close friend, particularly well-meaning advice that may work with neurotypical children but not children with ADHD.

Providing up-to-date, helpful resources that align with your approach to parenting a child with ADHD can make a significant difference in how others receive and respond to your child. Share articles, books, or reputable websites that explain ADHD in an accessible way. For example, you can direct them to Dr. Sharon Saline's excellent webpage on ADHD resources, which offers valuable insights into ADHD and family dynamics. Resources like these can help your extended family and friends understand ADHD better and support your child in more informed ways.

Conversely, know that this suggestion is for ideal circumstances. Even if you have incredibly caring and involved family members, they may not, through lack of time or interest, for example, follow up in examining any of your suggested resources. (If you think having shorter, more humorous resources would help, try passing along some of those in the following list instead.)

Simple and Helpful ADHD Resources

Here are a few scientifically grounded, accessible, dare we say even a little humorous, YouTube and other video resources that can help extended family members, coaches, and others better understand ADHD:

https://www.youtube.com/watch?v=J-AU_P4E27E (A news interview with Penn and Kim Holderness re: Penn's ADHD diagnosis and their book, *ADHD is Awesome*).

https://www.youtube.com/watch?v=ji0hg1LduU8 (This is What it's Really Like to Have ADHD: Interview snips explaining what it is like to have ADHD).

https://www.youtube.com/c/howtoadhd (How to ADHD. Have ADHD? Know someone with ADHD? Want to learn more? This channel is a great place to start).

https://www.youtube.com/watch?v=UmEpGaEUOqE&t=5s (Why ADHD is Like Having a Ferrari Brain with Bicycle Brakes, Dr. Edward Hallowell).

https://www.youtube.com/c/ADHDDudeRyanWexelblattLCSW (Fyan Wexelblatt's ADHD Dude channel offers many shorter and longer video resources).

If you are just starting on your journey of parenting a child with ADHD, it is unlikely you'll have a complete understanding of the condition (We, in fact, are still on that learning curve!). It may be hard to pull solid information, helpful facts, and anecdotal stories up at the drop of a hat.

Instead, just like you may role-play with your child with ADHD around communication with a teacher, practice a short statement explaining ADHD that you have handy to pull out as needed. Something in your own words. If we were explaining ADHD, it would include these details and sound something like this:

Children with ADHD often experience delays in emotional regulation and behavioral development, typically lagging behind their peers by several years in these areas. Research suggests this delay is due to differences in brain development, particularly in the prefrontal cortex, which is responsible for executive functions like impulse control, emotional regulation, and decision-making. That's why you see our child often exhibit impulsive actions, may be the brunt of their seemingly out-of-line emotional outbursts, or find them choosing poor verbal or physical behaviors. For example, a 10-year-old child with ADHD may exhibit emotional or behavioral responses more typical of a 7-year-old. This delay does not reflect a lack of intelligence or potential but rather a difference in the maturation of neural pathways.

What can you come up with that makes sense to you and is in your communication style?

Passing information along these lines can help relatives, coaches, tutors, and caregivers set realistic expectations and adopt strategies that support your child's developmental trajectory while fostering patience and resilience.

Then again, unfortunately, it may not. Interested parties may still believe that ADHD is "not a thing" or that your child is simply misbehaving and needs stricter parenting.

In that case, know that with all the tasks on your "parenting a child with ADHD plate," a) it is likely not possible for you to single-handedly transfer a helpful depth of knowledge to family and friends, b) nor will you necessarily have the energy to do so, and c) as a mom of a child with ADHD reminded us, nor do you have the responsibility to do so.

Therefore, setting boundaries is another crucial aspect of these interactions. It's essential to communicate your needs clearly and assertively. Let your family and friends who are interested know how they can support you and your child without overstepping. If you are at the beginning of your journey with ADHD, these boundaries will likely change over time, both as your child grows and as your understanding of their version of ADHD deepens. This will be an ongoing conversation.

Involving extended family and friends in family activities can, though, foster a broader support network. Invite them to participate in events where your child feels comfortable and supported. This involvement strengthens family bonds and provides your child with a wider circle of support, making them feel loved and understood in a broader context.

If conflicts arise, try to address them calmly and constructively. Use "I" statements to express your feelings and encourage open dialogue. For instance, "I feel overwhelmed when there's criticism about our parenting approach. Can we talk about how we can better support each other?" This approach fosters understanding and cooperation.

Empowering Your Child to Self-Advocate

Teaching self-advocacy skills to your child with ADHD is like giving them additional tools in their toolkit for navigating the world.

For example, concerning education, as they grow older, help them understand their rights, such as the right to accommodations in school under laws like—for those in the United States—the Individuals with Disabilities Education Act (IDEA). Explain what accommodations they are entitled to and how these can help them thrive in the school system. Encourage them to communicate their needs clearly and confidently.

Role-playing exercises can be a fun and practical way to teach self-advocacy. Set up scenarios where your child can practice asking for what they need. You can role-play being their teacher or soccer coach, and they can practice requesting a break or additional help with an assignment or drill.

Building confidence is crucial for effective self-advocacy. Start by celebrating small wins to boost their self-esteem. Positive reinforcement can go a long way in helping them feel capable and empowered. Involve them in decision-making processes, such as planning their study schedule or choosing extracurricular activities, as that engagement gives them a sense of control and ownership over their lives. Encourage them to set achievable goals and celebrate when they meet them. Confidence grows with each success, no matter how small.

TRAVELER ASSISTANCE

I (Alicia) have used a technique to improve dialogue with others that I learned from one of my mentors, Callan Rush. I call it the "I Imagine" technique.

It's simply a short dialogue that encourages the other person to start sharing their feelings, which might be a struggle for children with ADHD.

- Start with **"I see ..."** This is a true statement, as far as you can see. For example, "I see you drinking a glass of water."

- Then say, **"I imagine ..."** You are the only person who can imagine this; the other person is not imagining the same as you. For example, "I imagine you will feel calmer when you are hydrated."

- Then say, **"I am feeling ..."** You can express how you are feeling now, such as, "I am happy that you are hydrated." Here, it is essential to understand that you will not be able to know what the other person is feeling.

- And end with, **"Is this true?"**

Now, it is your turn to be quiet and listen to the other person's response.

Try it in any situation to understand what other people are feeling. It could be your child with ADHD, their sibling, or anybody else.

REST STOP

It's time for parents to take a break and digest information! Take 10 minutes of calm to Rest with the following questions:

1. **Reflect on sibling relationships:** How has ADHD in your family impacted sibling dynamics? Can you think of ways to foster understanding and reduce any resentment between siblings, ensuring a stronger sense of unity?

2. **Explore parental emotional health:** How do the demands of parenting a child with ADHD affect your emotional state and energy levels as a parent? Could making space for your emotional well-being improve the overall dynamics in your family?

Next, Stop for 10 minutes of quiet (sitting or slowly walking). Keep your mind as clear and open as possible, and just listen. Jot down or tell Siri to "make a note" of any responses that may arise. Because you've taken time to ponder calmly and quietly, these responses will most likely be less off-the-cuff and from a deeper level. They can give you clues as to the reasons behind your answers! Those clues, in turn, will reveal potential problematic thinking and can provide great direction on moving forward with the recommendations in this chapter that would be the easiest to implement or fit best for your family!

ROADWORK

Completing the Stress Cycle

Our Roadwork for this chapter is having your family grow in its understanding of completing the stress cycle as an effective tool for helping all family members manage stress.

This concept builds on the General Adaptation Syndrome (GAS) model proposed by Hans Selye, which outlines the body's three-stage response to stress. Many papers and books expand on this concept, but we'll focus on the work done by Emily Nagoski and Amelia Nagoski in their recent book, *Burnout: The Secret to Unlocking the Stress Cycle.*

Completing the stress cycle involves resolving the physiologic stress response and returning to balance to avoid long-term physical and mental harm. While the sources we mentioned provide a more thorough explanation, here's a brief overview of the stages and some practical strategies for completing the cycle.

1. **Alarm Stage:** This is the initial reaction to a stressor, during which the sympathetic nervous system activates the fight-or-flight, freeze-or-fawn response. Adrenaline and cortisol flood the bloodstream, increasing heart rate, breathing, muscle tension, and alertness.

2. **Resistance Stage:** After the immediate threat has passed, the parasympathetic nervous system (rest and relax) kicks in, helping the body regain balance. This stage might follow everyday stressors like school challenges or social interactions for children.

3. **Exhaustion Stage:** If the stress cycle isn't completed, persistent activation can lead to burnout, as described by Selye and echoed in the Nagoskis' work. Prolonged stress without release impairs the body's ability to cope, potentially leading to mental and physical health issues.

Completing the stress cycle is particularly essential for children with ADHD, as they are more prone to remaining in a heightened state of arousal. For example, children with a variant in the FKBP5 gene may experience over-activation of the HPA axis (which regulates cortisol), making it difficult for their cortisol levels to return to normal after a stressor. This cortisol dysregulation contributes to ongoing symptoms such as impulsivity, hyperactivity, and emotional dysregulation.

The impact of chronic stress is multifaceted:

- **Impaired Executive Functioning:** Elevated stress hormones like cortisol can impair cognitive functions, making tasks like focus and self-regulation more challenging.

- **Sleep Disruption:** Persistent stress disrupts sleep, which can further exacerbate ADHD symptoms.

- **Emotional Dysregulation:** Children with ADHD may seek instant gratification or "dopamine boosts," which, under stress, can lead to increased impulsivity or emotional outbursts.

Teaching your child to complete the stress cycle is crucial for emotional and behavioral regulation.

Years ago, I (Brenda) first learned of the way many animals will de-stress with physical movement; witness dogs shaking themselves dry after an unexpected dip in the water, horses bucking in an unfamiliar situation, and antelopes continuing to run, even after a predator has stopped chasing them. While those examples can be fun and simple ways to explain stress cycle completion to a young child, from Amelia and Emily Nagoski, I learned several other practices that, alongside shaking, bucking, and running, can be helpful endpoints for your child's body to know stress has passed, and they can calm and relax.

- **Mindful breathing:** Refer to the suggestions for different types of breathing in previous Steps. The Physiological Sigh, in particular, can activate the parasympathetic nervous system and let the body know it can come out of a stress response.

- **Physical activity:** Refer to Step Two – Move. Safe roughhousing, running around the backyard, and climbing playground apparatus are all helpful ways to discharge excess energy.

- **Creative outlets:** Refer to numerous RoadWorks activities and any other creative activities you have found that help your child release emotional tension.

- **Positive social connection:** Refer to the ADHD Family Dynamics section and consider ways to interact socially (e.g., taking a walk together or going on a tea date).

- **Affection:** Use positive physical touch with your child (e.g., massage and hugs). This releases oxytocin, which sends the child's brain the message that they are safe and can turn off the stress response.

- **Laughter:** It needs to be genuine, but if so, laughter can release tension and promote relaxation

- **Crying:** Allowing your child to cry can be a powerful way for them to complete the stress cycle. It doesn't need to be long, and it is most effective when they aren't dwelling on the preceding stressor while crying. However, it can be a great tool for releasing bottled-up stress.

And one more bonus method of completing the stress cycle?

- **Sound sleep:** Refer to the Sleep Step and implement tools to support your child's best rest, particularly deep (slow-wave) sleep and REM sleep, when the body processes and reduces stress hormones.

As a final note for this Roadwork, realize that children with ADHD often mimic the behaviors of those around them. Therefore, if you model any of the above stress cycle completion activities, your child may be responsive to modeling that behavior (behavioral mirroring). If you want your child to settle easier at bedtime, spend the evening quietening, yawning, lying beside your child, or wrapping up in a quilt or weighted blanket. Your child may follow your lead and give their brain a "safety" message that dials down the stress hormones.

Each activity tells the body it's safe and time to unwind. By helping your child complete the stress cycle regularly, you can reduce the long-term impact of stress and improve their emotional resilience.

SOUVENIR

This chapter's souvenir is giving yourself the gift of an hour of time.

An Hour of "Me Time" for Parents

As a parent of a child with ADHD, your days are likely packed with, among other things, managing schedules, navigating emotional roller coasters, responding to messages from daycare or school, getting educational accommodations in place, finding foods your child will eat, and ensuring your child feels supported and understood. But amid all this, carving out at least an hour for yourself every week is crucial. And by this, we aren't talking about grocery shopping, house cleaning, or driving to lessons or sports practices.

Here are three reasons why alone and non-task-based time is vital:

1. **Recharge Your Emotional Batteries:** While there are many unique delights in parenting a child with ADHD, it can also be extremely emo-

tionally draining. Taking an hour allows you to decompress and regain emotional balance, helping you stay patient and resilient in those more challenging moments.

2. **Maintain Your Own Identity:** It's easy to lose sight of your needs and passions when your focus is constantly on supporting your child to be best understood and flourish. Having alone time helps you reconnect with what makes you feel fulfilled and reminds you that you're more than a parent.

3. **Model Healthy Self-Care:** By prioritizing self-care, you teach your children the importance of caring for themselves and giving them examples. This shows them that everyone, including parents, deserves rest and time to recharge.

Ways to Carve Out an Hour:

1. **Swap Time with a Friend:** Find a trusted friend who also needs a break and agree to take turns watching each other's children for an hour each week. This way, both of you can enjoy some personal time while knowing your kids are in good hands and potentially enjoying a playdate.

2. **Enlist Family Support:** Ask a grandparent, sibling, or other family member to spend time with your child. Even if it's just once a week, this regular break can give you time to yourself while allowing your child to bond with other important people.

3. **Use Evening Time:** Consider using the first hour after your child goes to bed for some dedicated "me time." Instead of immediately finishing kitchen tidying or tackling some of your work or self-employed tasks, make it a "me time." Whether reading a book, enjoying a bath, or journaling, schedule a peaceful time to unwind.

Finding that hour each week might take some planning and might not work out every week. But when possible, the benefits to your well-being—and ultimately, your ability to support your child—make it absolutely worth it.

Finally, in our last chapter, we'll explore medical and alternative treatments, providing a holistic view of how to further support your child's unique needs.

Chapter 13

Supplemental Essentials Three - Medical and Alternative Treatments

"The art of healing comes from nature, not from the physician. Therefore, the physician must start from nature, with an open mind."

- Paracelsus, author of Die Grosse Wundartzney

S UMMARY - Travel Size Version

To say navigating the world of ADHD treatments can be overwhelming is a bit of an understatement. Truthfully, it can sometimes feel like you're finding your way out of a never-ending, no-direction-provided maze.

This Step will cover critical points related to therapy and medical treatments and review supplement options in clear, easy-to-understand language. The maze won't be eliminated, but hopefully, you'll have tools to shed some light on the journey.

Behavioral Therapy

First, we'll briefly recap and then expand on the concept of behavioral therapy. We have mentioned CBT several times, but we want to give you a few other therapy suggestions focusing on behavior modification and social skills training. We'll also briefly compare behavioral therapy and attachment parenting and suggest a hybrid model.

Medications and Medication Side Effects

In our scope of practice, we don't diagnose or treat disease states or prescribe medication. We can, however, provide some understanding of how certain ADHD medications work and how some of their effects may be impacted by different gene codings related to dopamine and serotonin genes, as well as inflammation, detoxification, and stress genes.

In this section, we'll also provide some clues about potential side effects.

Natural Supplements and Their Role in ADHD Treatment

Natural supplements can be a valuable addition to your child's treatment plan. We'll recap our favorites here.

Treatment Plan Changes

Sometimes, despite your best efforts, the current treatment plan you are using for your child with ADHD might not be working as well as you'd hoped. Consult with your healthcare providers and invite them to guide you through exploring alternative options, whether trying a different medication or adding complementary therapies like mindfulness practices or neurofeedback.

Note, too, that the seven Core Steps outlined in this book are a great place to start and provide an excellent framework for any other treatment considerations you decide to make.

Finally, remember that transitioning to a new treatment plan—especially one that includes a change in medications or dosages—should always be done gradually and under medical supervision to ensure its safety and effectiveness.

INFORMATION CENTER

It's 8:00 PM, and your house is still a flurry of activity. You're trying to get lunches made for the next day and ensure backpacks are primed and ready to go. Your youngest child, who has ADHD, is bouncing around, struggling to focus on getting PJs on and prepared for bed. You've tried every parenting hack in the book, but the whole family is on edge. Your predominant thought? "Is there something out there that could help my child manage their symptoms better?"

Behavioral Therapy: Techniques and Outcomes

Behavioral therapy, an overarching term for a range of therapies that treat mental and emotional health disorders, has as its premise the belief that behaviors are learned and that behaviors can be changed.

Using one or more types of behavioral therapy (e.g., CBT, Cognitive Behavioral Play Therapy, behavior modification, Dialectical Behavioral Therapy, Acceptance, and Commitment Therapy) can be a very effective strategy in your parenting toolkit. In most cases, particularly when a child is very young or unwilling to attend therapy sessions, many of these forms of behavioral therapy can be very effective for parents, which, in turn, means they are helpful for their children.

At its foundation, behavioral therapy consists of several components designed to help your child manage ADHD symptoms more effectively. These include behavior modification, cognitive-behavioral therapy (CBT), and social skills training.

- **Behavior modification** focuses on identifying triggers for certain behaviors and implementing strategies to encourage positive actions while reducing negative ones.

- **CBT** helps children understand the connections between their thoughts, feelings, and behaviors, equipping them with tools to challenge and change unhelpful thought patterns.

- **Social skills training** teaches children how to interact appropriately with others, fostering better relationships and reducing social anxiety.

Together, these approaches can empower your child to navigate situations where their ADHD brain may not naturally align with environmental expectations. Specific techniques such as positive reinforcement, time management training, and problem-solving skills are actionable tools for improvement. For example, rewarding desirable behavior—like offering extra Lego-building time for completing homework—encourages its recurrence. Breaking tasks into smaller steps with timers helps children stay on track, and problem-solving skills teach them to evaluate options and choose effective solutions. These methods improve immediate behavior and lay the foundation for lifelong coping strategies.

While these techniques might involve navigating initial challenges—like filling the odd hole in the wall or reinforcing consistent consequences—you can anticipate significant improvements in your child's behavior, emotional regulation, and social interactions. The goal is not to stifle the unique and creative aspects of an ADHD brain but to foster a more harmonious household with fewer meltdowns and more positive engagement.

Behavioral Therapy, Attachment Parenting, and a Suggested Hybrid

For some parents, behavioral modification as a primary approach can feel overly rigid. They may gravitate toward some variation of attachment parenting, which emphasizes building a strong emotional connection with the child. Practices like responsive caregiving, co-sleeping, and breastfeeding aim to meet a child's emotional and physical needs, fostering self-regulation and reducing anxiety.

Attachment parenting can be particularly effective for children with ADHD, who are often misunderstood. A secure parent-child bond can reduce stress and improve emotional stability. However, it may lack tools to address ADHD's immediate behavioral challenges, such as impulsivity or aggression. Additionally, the high parental involvement required can lead to caregiver burnout, especially with higher-needs children.

Instead of focusing solely on one parenting style, we suggest parents ask, *"What kind of parenting does my child need right now?"* This approach allows for flexibility and addresses the ever-changing needs of children with ADHD. A hybrid model, integrating behavioral therapy strategies with attachment parenting, can be particularly effective.

The Effective Parenting model provides a helpful framework. It identifies three types of children—each with strengths and challenges—and the parenting styles that best meet their needs. While every parent embodies aspects of all these styles and every child demonstrates a mix of these behavioral patterns, the key lies in recognizing which approach is most effective at a given moment. This flexibility allows parents to adapt to their child's temperament while providing the tools and support necessary to navigate ADHD.

The Force Child and the Mentor Parent

Force children are strong-willed, passionate, and driven by intense emotions—for Star Wars fans think the "Force" is strong with this one! While their energy and creativity can be assets, they often struggle with impulsivity and frustration.

- **Strengths of a Force Child**: Force children are natural leaders and innovators. They excel when their energy is channeled into constructive outlets.

- **Challenges with ADHD**: Their intensity can amplify impulsivity and defiance, making them prone to outbursts and power struggles, particularly when faced with rules they find unfair.

The Mentor Parent provides a mix of empathy, patience, and clear boundaries. This style focuses on guiding rather than controlling. Mentor parents can:

- Validate the child's big emotions without overreacting, offering tools for self-regulation.

- Set firm but flexible boundaries that provide structure while ensuring the child feels heard.

- Encourage constructive energy use through collaboration and natural consequences instead of punishment.

When guided by a Mentor parent, Force children's bold nature becomes a great strength, fostering self-regulation, decision-making, and confidence.

The Cooperation Child and the Team Parent

Cooperation children thrive in collaborative, inclusive environments. They are naturally social, adaptable, and motivated by teamwork.

- **Strengths of a Cooperation Child**: They excel in group activities, demonstrate strong communication skills, and value connection.

- **Challenges with ADHD**: They may struggle with impulsivity or distractibility in social settings and feel sidelined if perceived as "different." Their desire to please can lead to emotional burnout or stress when expectations aren't met.

The Team Parent works alongside the Cooperation child, fostering mutual respect and collaboration. For ADHD parenting, this means balancing partnership with guidance. Team parents can:

- Encourage problem-solving together (e.g., "What can we do to make this easier? What would you do, in this case, to solve this problem?").

- Act as a supportive coach, focusing on effort rather than outcomes.

- Create a cooperative family dynamic where all voices are heard, but the parent remains the ultimate guide.

This approach empowers Cooperation children to thrive socially while building confidence in navigating ADHD-related challenges.

The Security Child and the Willpower Parent

Security children thrive on structure, predictability, and reassurance. They are highly sensitive and may struggle in chaotic environments or with big emotions.

- **Strengths of a Security Child**: Empathetic, thoughtful, and detail-oriented, they excel in settings where they feel safe and supported.

- **Challenges with ADHD**: These children may be overwhelmed by sensory stimuli, frequent anxiety, or resistance to change, leading to meltdowns or withdrawal.

The Willpower Parent provides the clear boundaries and consistent routines Security children need to feel secure. For ADHD parenting, this requires balancing firmness with compassion. Willpower parents can:

- Create predictable routines to reduce anxiety.

- Communicate transitions clearly to prepare the child for change.

- Set and uphold boundaries while remaining emotionally sensitive.

This approach helps Security children develop resilience and confidence, ensuring they feel supported even amid ADHD-related challenges.

Behavioral Model

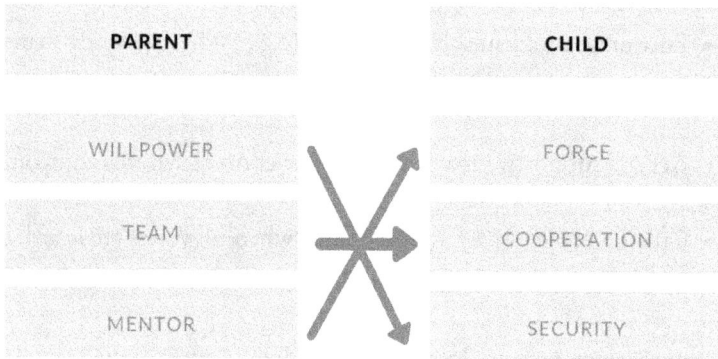

PARENT		CHILD
WILLPOWER		FORCE
TEAM		COOPERATION
MENTOR		SECURITY

From: Effective Parenting, Niños de Ahora, Mexico

Blending Approaches for ADHD

Understanding your child's behavioral style allows you to adjust your parenting approach to meet their needs in the moment. Security children may need Willpower parents to provide stability, while Cooperation children thrive with Team parents who foster connection. Force children benefit most from Mentor parents who balance guidance with empathy.

The last thing a Force child needs is a Willpower parent. This combination may create an unstable environment where things are most likely not appropriately managed. It may also result in rivalry between the child and the parent instead of finding answers.

A hybrid approach—integrating attachment parenting's emotional foundation with the behavioral strategies of the Effective Parenting model—offers a robust parenting framework. For example:

- Use a healthy parent-child attachment to build trust and reduce anxiety.

- Shift to Mentor parenting during challenging moments to provide structure and guidance.

This synergy delivers emotional safety alongside actionable tools for managing ADHD-related behaviors.

By combining emotional connection, structure, and practical strategies and using various combinations of those skills to match their child's needs at any given point, parents can create a holistic approach tailored to their child's unique challenges and strengths. This flexibility fosters resilience, confidence, and harmony in navigating the complexities of ADHD.

Medications for ADHD: Types, Benefits, and Mechanism of Action

When it comes to treating ADHD, medications can often play a crucial role. For some children, the benefits of these medications can be quite transformative. There are two main types of medications used with ADHD: stimulants and non-stimulants.

- Stimulant medications like amphetamines and methylphenidate work by increasing dopamine and norepinephrine levels in the brain. These neurotransmitters are integral for attention, focus, and impulse control. They enhance concentration and reduce impulsivity and hyperactivity.

- Non-stimulants, on the other hand, primarily stabilize norepinephrine levels, making them a suitable option for children who may not respond well to stimulants. Thus, they aid in better impulse control and focus without the intensity of stimulant effects.

I (Alicia) remember a mom of a child with ADHD sharing that her son didn't eat much during the day while his medication was active, but later, as the medication wore off, he would become very hungry. This is a common side effect of stimulant medications because dopamine plays a crucial role in the brain's reward system, which includes regulating hunger. Elevated dopamine levels during medication use can reduce the brain's drive to seek food, making the body more satisfied.

Stimulant medications also activate the sympathetic nervous system, triggering the body's fight-or-flight response. In this state, the body prioritizes alertness and readiness over digestion and hunger, suppressing appetite.

Another mechanism at play is the potential for stimulant medications to slow gastric emptying—the rate at which food leaves the stomach. This delay can make your child feel full for longer periods.

If your child's medication peaks during school hours or earlier in the day, it may explain why they do not feel hungry at those times. The appetite suppression is temporary, and hunger often returns as the medication wears off.

Suppose medication is part of your child's treatment plan. In that case, it's crucial to work with your healthcare provider to regularly monitor dosage and timing or consider switching to a non-stimulant ADHD medication if appetite suppression becomes a significant issue. Balanced meals remain essential for maintaining your child's energy levels and supporting growth. Prolonged undernutrition can negatively impact both.

Other potential side effects of ADHD medications include fatigue, increased activity levels, mood swings (especially as the medication wears off), anxiety, tics, upset stomach, sleep disturbances, and changes in blood pressure or heart rate. These should also be monitored and discussed with your healthcare provider to ensure your child's well-being.

Note, too, that it may take time for healthcare providers to be able to appropriately prescribe an effective drug, as it is a trial-and-error process.

However, are medications truly necessary or beneficial for everyone diagnosed with ADHD?

In short, not always. Not everyone with an ADHD diagnosis requires medication. Knowing if your child is a candidate is best discussed with their healthcare provider and balanced with your knowledge of your child, potential side effects of different medications, and from where you may be getting "medicate" messages.

As Dr. Maté mentions in his book *Scattered Minds*, in many cases, it is the school system that subtly or not so subtly puts pressure on parents to give medications to their children (with no slams on our part on overworked teachers lacking the resources to deal with days filled with situational mismatches!). In that case, they likely see behaviors they think the medication would help—behaviors potentially interfering with the child's learning.

While we are not saying whether or not this advice should be followed (remember, nutritionists don't diagnose or treat), parents should work with the school to address these concerns (e.g., the treatments and tools they use at home and how they can collaborate with the school). We suggest that you consider a wide range of information, including how medications interact with your child's genetics when deciding whether to proceed with medication.

Common ADHD Medications

Medication	Duration	Common Side Effects	Mechanism of Action
Ritalin (Methylphenidate) (Stimulant)	Short-acting (3-4 hours)	Decreased appetite, trouble sleeping, headache	Blocks dopamine and norepinephrine reuptake, increasing levels in the brain
Concerta (Methylphenidate) (Stimulant)	Extended-release (10-12 hours)	Decreased appetite, irritability, difficulty sleeping	Blocks dopamine and norepinephrine reuptake, increasing levels in the brain with a sustained release
Adderall (Amphetamine) (Stimulant)	Immediate-release (4-6 hours), XR (10-12 hours)	Increased heart rate, anxiety, appetite loss	Promotes release and blocks reuptake of dopamine and norepinephrine
Vyvanse (Lisdexamfetamine) (Stimulant)	Extended-release (10-14 hours)	Dry mouth, insomnia, irritability	Prodrug converted to dextroamphetamine, promoting dopamine and norepinephrine release and blocking reuptake
Atomoxetine (Non-Stimulant)	Extended-release (24 hours)	Upset stomach, fatigue, mood swings	Selective norepinephrine reuptake inhibitor, increasing norepinephrine levels in the brain
Intuniv (Guanfacine) (Non-Stimulant	Extended-release (24 hours)	Drowsiness, dizziness, dry mouth	Alpha-2A adrenergic receptor agonist, reducing sympathetic nerve impulses and improving attention

Dopamine's Negative Feedback Loop

Stimulants commonly used to treat ADHD work by preventing the reuptake of dopamine into the presynaptic neuron, causing an increase in dopamine levels in the synaptic cleft. These effects enhance dopaminergic signaling, improving attention and behavioral control, which underscores the central role of dopamine in the neurobiology of ADHD. To fully understand how stimulants impact dopamine signaling, it's essential to consider the negative feedback loop that regulates dopamine levels and activity.

The negative feedback loop for dopamine is a regulatory mechanism that helps maintain balance in dopamine signaling. It's not necessarily triggered only by "too much" dopamine in the synapse but by the system's ongoing monitoring of dopamine activity to prevent excessive or insufficient signaling. Here's how it works:

1. **Dopamine Release and Binding:** Dopamine is released into the synaptic cleft and binds to receptors on the postsynaptic neuron to transmit its signal. The DRD2 SNP plays a role in determining how well the dopamine receptors function.

2. **Dopamine Reuptake:** Some dopamine molecules bind to autoreceptors on the presynaptic neuron, acting as dopamine level sensors. The DAT1 SNP influences how effectively dopamine is reuptaken into the presynaptic neuron for recycling or breakdown.

3. **Signal Regulation:**

   ○ If dopamine levels in the presynaptic neuron are sufficient or excessive, a signal is sent to that neuron to reduce further dopamine production. This is the negative feedback loop in action, preventing overstimulation.

   ○ If dopamine levels in the presynaptic neuron are too low, this neuron will increase dopamine production. This is the negative feedback loop in action, promoting stimulation.

4. **Enzymatic Breakdown:** The role of enzymes like COMT (refer to the COMT SNP) adds to this interplay. These enzymes regulate how quickly dopamine is broken down or not, further impacting the overall availability of dopamine in the brain.

Together, these SNPs demonstrate the complexity of the dopaminergic pathways. Introducing medications, which often alter dopamine levels or signaling mechanisms, adds another layer to this complexity. Understanding your child's unique genetic profile can help predict how their brain responds to dopamine regulation and provide insights into the potential side effects of medication.

This is the beauty of integrating genetic insights into the everyday management of ADHD. By "marrying" genetic knowledge with how your child naturally handles dopamine and its receptors, you can better navigate challenges. Whether it involves adjusting lifestyle strategies or carefully monitoring medication, this understanding empowers you to make more informed and personalized decisions.

Why This Matters in ADHD

In ADHD, issues like impaired dopamine receptor function (e.g., DRD2 variations), dopamine reuptake, or altered autoreceptor sensitivity (e.g., DAT1 variations) can disrupt this feedback mechanism.

To sum up, the negative feedback loop is a finely tuned process that balances dopamine availability to ensure optimal neurotransmitter signaling. In ADHD brains, it is impaired and has difficulty maintaining balance. Medications for ADHD often target this imbalance by modulating dopamine reuptake to compensate for irregularities. However, this is generally targeted by trial and error between medications and dosages.

How Many ADHD Medications Work

Many ADHD medications work by increasing dopamine levels in the brain through blocking its reuptake. Why is this important? Because this mechanism interacts with the brain's negative feedback system. Usually, dopamine reuptake sends a signal back to the presynaptic neuron, effectively saying, "There's enough dopamine, no need to produce more." When reuptake is blocked, this message doesn't get delivered. As a result, the presynaptic neuron assumes it needs to produce more dopamine, amplifying the signaling. It's as if the neuron is saying, "More, more!"

This increased dopamine can help the brain with concentration, but conversely, that is why a potential side effect of these medications can be trouble sleeping or not being hungry. It is like turning on your space heater, full blast day and night.

The following figure illustrates how blocking dopamine reuptake works. The diagram outlines the presynaptic and postsynaptic neurons and the three SNPs we've discussed that influence dopamine pathways. Most stimulant medications block dopamine reuptake into the presynaptic neuron by interacting with the DAT1 SNP. This action increases dopamine levels in the synaptic cleft (the space between neurons), allowing DRD2 receptors on the postsynaptic neuron to receive more dopamine and enhance signaling.

Simultaneously, blocking DAT1 reduces dopamine levels in the presynaptic neuron, preventing it from receiving the usual feedback message, "There's enough dopamine; slow production." This lack of feedback prompts the presynaptic neuron to ramp up dopamine production, which improves focus and motivation.

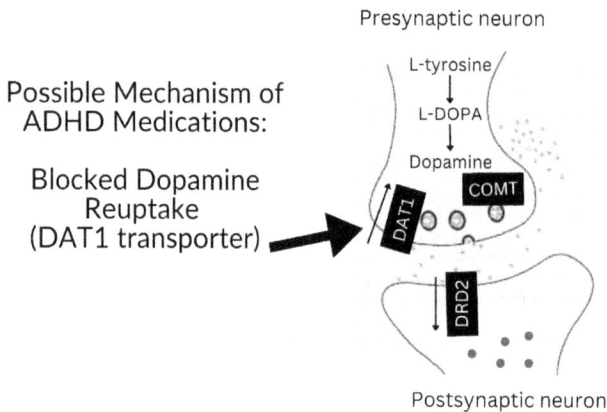

Possible Mechanism of ADHD Medications:

Blocked Dopamine Reuptake (DAT1 transporter)

Presynaptic neuron

L-tyrosine
L-DOPA
Dopamine
COMT
DAT1
DRD2

Postsynaptic neuron

Medications, Dopamine Genes and Possible Scenarios

This section examines the genetics of ADHD and how our dopamine SNPs may interact with medications. We will discuss possible case scenarios, especially those concentrating on the COMT, DRD2, and DAT1 genes.

I (Alicia) am variant for the COMT gene. This means I don't break down dopamine, norepinephrine, or epinephrine and, in turn, have high dopamine levels. These elevated dopamine levels are the primary reason I have trouble falling asleep. My DRD2 is heterozygous, meaning about 50% of the dopamine that gets into the neuron cleft makes it to the next neuron. For me, if I were taking medication for ADHD, it would most likely aggravate my situation rather than help.

A 9-year-old boy diagnosed with ADHD and with the same coding for COMT and DRD2 as Alicia was given a stimulant medication. For the parents, the increased hyperactivity seen after only two days on the stimulant medication was enough for his parents to know it was not going to work for him.

Rachel, however, is normal for COMT. This means that she constantly breaks down dopamine, norepinephrine, and epinephrine. Although she might be more "chilled" than me in terms of stress, her ADHD would likely benefit from medication. Although her DRD2 is green, and most dopamine makes it to the receptors, her dopamine levels are low.

In another and more challenging scenario, let's look at someone who is a normal COMT (easily and constantly breaking down dopamine, norepinephrine, or epinephrine) and variant DRD2 (makes less dopamine and has less getting to receptors). In this instance, the person would need a lot of dopamine for some to make it to the next cell. These children and adults would, in general, highly benefit from promoting dopamine synthesis by taking the correct supplement, implementing relevant lifestyle changes, such as daily exercise, and talking with an ADHD-focused health practitioner regarding medication.

These COMT effects are why the Goldilocks position for COMT, regarding its work with dopamine and stress hormones like epinephrine and norepinephrine, is heterozygous. You don't break down too much dopamine, but you also break down some stress hormones. Also, it would be optimal to be normal for DRD2, as then you are making sufficient amounts of dopamine and efficiently transmitting its messages to the next neuron.

In an ideal world, it would be nice if we all had that gene coding, but that is obviously not the case. The fact that we're all genetically different and have varying environmental influences is a factor in why, for some people like me (Alicia), a medication of this type would not be helpful, whereas, for others like Rachel, it might be OK. These differences can also be a factor in why, as Dr.

Maté explains, in many cases, the medications don't work, and they could cause unpleasant side effects like headaches, loss of appetite, listlessness, insomnia, or anxiety.

ADHD Medication Side Effects

Like any medication, those used for ADHD come with potential side effects. As mentioned, the most common are insomnia and loss of appetite, with insomnia potentially caused by an extra-stimulation of too much dopamine and appetite dysregulation potentially because of the interaction between dopamine and ghrelin (think back to our FTO reference in Step Three – Eat and this gene's influence on neural pathways regulating reward processing and appetite).

Anxiety, nervousness, headaches, irritability, or mood swings are also common. Some children might experience tics, growth delays, gastrointestinal issues, fatigue, or even more severe side effects like suicidal thoughts or liver damage. Non-stimulant medications also have their share of side effects, including dry mouth, skin reactions, and potential liver toxicity. When deciding on a treatment plan for your child, a medication's possible side effects are an essential consideration.

Monitoring and managing these medications require a vigilant approach. Regular follow-ups with your healthcare provider are essential to adjust dosages and address side effects. If you notice any adverse effects, it's important to communicate these promptly to your child's doctor. They may recommend adjusting the dosage or trying a different medication.

Genetic factors, such as variations in the CYP genes (see more information on this in Step Five – Detox), can also influence how your child metabolizes these medications, affecting their efficacy and side effects. Understanding these genetic influences can guide more personalized and effective treatment plans.

As with other wellness facets you have been monitoring with your child, such as sleep, movement, food, and mood, if your child is on medication, it is also important to keep a medication monitoring journal (see this Step's Roadwork for an example). A journal will help you keep a diligent record should any side effects begin to appear.

As mentioned, ADHD medications often work by inhibiting the dopamine reuptake process. They focus on the DAT1 SNP, helping to maintain dopamine levels in the synaptic cleft. For some children with ADHD on dopamine-increasing medications, there is a constant excess of dopamine in the interneuron space. This excess dopamine is then metabolized into norepinephrine and epinephrine via the normal process of maintaining appropriate dopamine levels.

When this occurs, the excess norepinephrine and epinephrine in the brain increases stress, anxiety, and irritability (affecting the ability to respond calmly or engage with new activities, among others) and can significantly disrupt your child's sleep patterns. This can be particularly challenging when it's bedtime for your child who is on this type of medication. Instead of being able to sleep, they seek more dopamine, often via small "winning events" such as getting likes or comments on social media or playing a video game, or via more challenging behaviors such as irritating a sibling or trying to start an argument with a parent.

In our discussions with Dr. Kendall-Reed about ADHD, her concern is that, in many instances today, we are giving a child's brain too much dopamine, whether from food, medication, or activities like video games. Think of this overly heightened sensation as too much of a dopaminergic surge, as it were. The excess dopamine can foster a phenomenon known as dopamine receptor downregulation (e.g., receptor downregulation—DRD2—and altered transporter activity—DAT1). This, in turn, can result in lower dopamine sensitivity, reduced baseline dopamine levels, and an escalation cycle of seeking more intense stimulation.

Another expert we hold in high regard, Dr. Robert Melillo, has suggested that stimulant medications may lose their effectiveness for some individuals over time. However, research indicates this is not a universal outcome and depends on factors like proper management and adherence. Dr. Melillo has also hypothesized that differences in activity between the brain's hemispheres may contribute to ADHD symptoms. He raises the question of whether current medications acting on the brain's overall neurotransmitter systems can precisely target the hemisphere that may require more dopamine support. While this area of research is still evolving, it highlights the complexity of ADHD treatment and the need for ongoing study into personalized approaches.

As Dr. Mate has expressed, "*Only one person has the right to decide whether a medication is taken: the one about to be treated.*" And "*The aim of medication is not to control behavior but to help children focus.*" Our caveat here would be that when the person about to be treated is a child who doesn't yet understand what is going on inside themselves, have the capacity to self-reflect or be able to emotionally regulate, the medication decision should be handled by a parent who best knows the child.

We are not psychologists or psychiatrists, nor, as stated previously, is prescribing medication within our scope of practice. We hope, however, that we have explained why medications for ADHD are not inherently good or bad. Instead, your specific genes can provide personalized guidelines for using medications. Those guidelines can provide a framework for discussion with your healthcare practitioners who can prescribe medications for ADHD.

What lies within our scope of practice is emphasizing the value of a holistic view. ADHD often involves a dopamine imbalance stemming from the interplay of multiple genes regulating dopamine levels and signaling. As we've seen throughout this book, lifestyle factors further complicate this process. This highlights the power of understanding your child's unique epigenetic roadmap.

While medications can address one aspect of this complex system, they are limited in scope. In contrast, the natural strategies outlined in this book address a broader range of genetic and environmental factors (e.g., the interplay between COMT, DRD2, and DAT1). As a foundational step, we recommend implementing these approaches to help balance dopamine levels, pairing them with additional recommendations for managing the challenging symptoms your child may be experiencing.

Serotonin and Attention-Deficit/Hyperactivity Disorder

The connection between serotonin and ADHD is less well-established than the role of dopamine and norepinephrine. Still, emerging research suggests that serotonin also plays a vital role in regulating mood, impulsivity, and attention, all of which are affected in ADHD.

Certain genetic polymorphisms in serotonin-related genes (such as 5-HTTL-PR, which affects serotonin reuptake transporter function) have been linked to

ADHD. Some studies have suggested that individuals with ADHD who carry specific variants of these genes may have alterations in serotonin signaling, which could contribute to symptoms of hyperactivity and impulsivity.

ADHD often coexists with other conditions, particularly anxiety and depression, which are heavily influenced by serotonin dysregulation. In these cases, serotonin imbalances may exacerbate ADHD symptoms, particularly emotional dysregulation and impulsivity.

Selective serotonin reuptake inhibitors (SSRIs), a class of antidepressants that target serotonin, are sometimes used in conjunction with stimulant medications to help manage mood disorders that frequently co-occur with ADHD.

In simple terms, while dopamine and norepinephrine remain the primary neurotransmitters associated with ADHD, serotonin also plays a role. Dysregulation of serotonin may contribute to the impulsive and hyperactive symptoms of ADHD, and it can also be relevant in cases where ADHD coexists with anxiety or depression. The serotonergic system may influence treatment outcomes, especially when managing emotional dysregulation and impulsivity in ADHD.

One significant fact is that about 90% of the body's serotonin is produced in the gastrointestinal (GI) tract. Dysbiosis—an imbalance in the gut's intestinal terrain—can negatively affect serotonin production. Conditions such as irritable bowel syndrome (IBS), inflammatory bowel disease (IBD), and other gastrointestinal disorders often show altered serotonin levels in the gut, which can contribute to symptoms such as abnormal gut motility, diarrhea, or constipation.

These serotonin disruptions in the gut can also have downstream effects on mood and cognitive function through the gut-brain axis. Is there a relationship between ADHD symptoms and our gut? Most likely, yes. That's another reason we must pay special attention to a child's digestive health.

As we have mentioned before and will continue to emphasize, an interplay of factors contributes to ADHD. The microbiome's health is essential for maintaining proper serotonin balance, which impacts not only gastrointestinal function but also mood and mental health through the gut-brain connection.

Though we haven't explicitly mentioned our microbiome—aside from suggesting many Eat recommendations that can support its balance—there is a SNP we can pay attention to here: the **FUT2** gene. This gene's effects on gut bacterial populations and mucosal health can impact how much serotonin is produced and how it is regulated within the gut environment.

Finally, and continuing the Eat theme, what about our dietary habits? We know that dopamine interacts with ghrelin. When dopamine is abnormal, it starts to increase ghrelin (the hunger hormone), which fosters the addictive pattern that those with ADHD can have with sugar. Following the recommendations in Step One – Eat can help stop the sugar-addiction cycle.

Medications and Inflammation, Detoxification, and Stress Genes

Why is it that when we "older folks" were kids, it seemed ADHD was virtually nonexistent? Have we evolved as a human species in only one or two generations to have problems with dopamine? Is this the reason why all of these medications focus on dopamine for ADHD? Or are there other contributing factors to the rapid onset of ADHD worldwide?

While improved diagnostic mechanisms, broader cultural awareness, and acceptance of mental health discussions may play a role, they may not fully explain the rise in diagnoses. According to Dr. Kendall-Reed, dopamine production and receptors have remained constant throughout generations.

If so, that means that to serve our children with ADHD best, we cannot only concentrate on neurotransmitters (which have stayed the same) and "treat" people with medications to deal with that aspect of health.

What about the other changes that have occurred in the world in a relatively short period? By concentrating on dopamine and medications, are we overlooking three critical changes in the world: inflammation, stress, and detoxification?

In Step Five – Detox, Step Six – Calm, and Step Seven – Inflammation, we mentioned that several genes in each category are worth paying attention to regarding ADHD symptoms.

The scientific literature, however, hasn't paid much attention to the relationship between ADHD medications and brain inflammation, possibly because the typical side effects of ADHD medications are not commonly associated with brain inflammation.

Research suggests, though, that inflammation can interfere with neural communication, including dopamine signaling, even when dopamine production and receptor function are intact. Chronic inflammation may disrupt the signal transmission between neurons, potentially exacerbating or mimicking ADHD symptoms. While more research is needed to understand how inflammation specifically interacts with dopamine pathways, these findings highlight the importance of addressing inflammation as part of ADHD management (i.e., review the information on the IL6 and TNF-α genes).

Likewise, with stress? It is well known that inflammation and stress negatively impact gene expression (i.e., cause our genes to behave as if they were in a less-than-helpful position). If a child has a constant cycle of stress and inflammation, where levels of both remain high, at that point, it doesn't matter how "good" their dopamine production and receptors are; the inflammation and stress will dictate what happens with health (i.e., review the information on the COMT, FKBP5, and GAD1 genes).

Sadly, the influence on ADHD symptoms doesn't end there. As most of us are well aware, the amount of toxins in the environment, food, air, and water today is alarming. Toxicity can lead to inflammation as the body's immune system responds to harmful substances. When toxic substances enter the body—whether through chemicals, pollutants, heavy metals, drugs, or even by-products of metabolism—the immune system recognizes them as harmful. It initiates an inflammatory response to neutralize and remove the toxins. Think back to Step Five – Detox. Is your child's liver metabolizing toxins, both those coming in from the environment and the internally produced natural by-products of activities such as exercise?

If you as a parent have decided to, for example, put your child on medication that increases dopamine for school days, then something you can perhaps pair with that is ensuring that both inflammation and stress are down during the days your child is on the medication.

Or, if you have chosen, in partnership with your health practitioners, to take your child off medication, our suggestion is to understand your child's genetic makeup and, again, in collaboration with your health practitioners, wean off any medication very slowly. Should your health practitioner agree, and dopamine production or regulation be an issue, a helpful supplement that can be used during and after that process is to have your child take the amino acid tyrosine, the dopamine precursor.

According to Dr. Andrew Huberman, neuroscientist and tenured professor in Stanford University's Department of Neurobiology, the addictive effects of ADHD medications occur, as per Dr. Kendall-Reed's observations, because overloading the brain with high levels of dopamine can lead to the downregulation of dopamine receptors or depletion of dopamine stores. As a result, users need increasingly higher doses to achieve the same effect.

Dr. Huberman also mentions that appropriately prescribed and safe drugs are a trial and error. If your child doesn't have any side effects from their use, they are probably getting the "ideal medication and dosage." In the real world, a mom told me (Alicia) that it has been at least three years of trial and error for her child without being able to avoid side effects and still seeing behavioral challenges.

Thus, we suggest understanding the interplay of your child's genetics in how they respond to stress, toxicity, and inflammation. By addressing the book's Core Steps, you may find an alternate solution or, at least, a helpful complement to stimulant medication.

Natural Supplements and Their Role in ADHD Support

Natural supplements can offer a range of benefits when managing ADHD. Throughout the book, we've touched on many different supplement options. Scientific evidence supports these:

- Tyrosine: dopamine precursor, improved focus and mood.

- Magnesium: supports relaxation and sleep.

- Omega-3 fatty acids: play a crucial role in brain function.

- Zinc: essential for neurotransmitter function and can help improve hyperactivity and impulsivity.

- 5-HTP: serotonin precursor; reduces symptoms of anxiety and depression.

- GABA and L-theanine: have calming properties that can help manage anxiety.

- N-acetyl-cysteine and Glutathione: support liver detoxification and inflammation.

- DIM: supports liver detoxification and metabolism.

- Lactium: reduces stress.

Keep in mind that several of these compounds can be found in food. For example, tyrosine can be used in supplement form. You can also find it in soybeans, chicken, turkey, fish, almonds, avocados, bananas, cheese, yogurt, chickpeas, pumpkin seeds, and sesame seeds.

It's important to note that while these supplements can be beneficial, they are not necessarily a substitute for traditional treatments and should be part of a comprehensive management plan. As we saw when we examined SNPs and medications, knowing your child's DNA is an excellent asset for selecting and adjusting supplements.

If you are considering using some of these supplements with your child, they are outlined in the Supplement Appendix. Remember that recommended dosages vary depending on the supplement and your child's age, weight, and individual needs based on DNA and life circumstances. For example, omega-3 fatty acid dosages typically range from 500 to 1,000 mg daily, while zinc supplements usually range from 5-10 mg daily. Therapeutic dosages of zinc for ADHD can range from 20-40 mg but under medical supervision. Magnesium supplements can vary from 100 to 300 mg daily, depending on the child's age and dietary intake.

In addition, make sure you check the quality control of any supplements you are considering purchasing. This Step's Traveler Assistance gives some good criteria to use, as, in the past, we have found that not all supplements are of the quality that will provide a positive outcome.

It's important to discuss any new supplements with a healthcare provider (e.g., doctor, pharmacist) to avoid potential interactions with medications, to ensure they are needed, and, if so, how much to take and when.

Monitoring the effectiveness of supplements is as good an idea as tracking the effectiveness of medications. It involves observing changes in behavior, attention, and overall mood. Keep a journal to track improvements and note any side effects. (Again, note a helpful log in this Step's Roadwork.)

Gastrointestinal issues, headaches, or changes in sleep patterns can be signs that a supplement may need to be adjusted or discontinued. Keep in mind, as well, that some supplements, such as Lactium, might take several weeks before their effectiveness begins to be felt. The first time I (Alicia) took Lactium, I thought it wasn't beneficial. Why? Because on the label, the directions state to take it with food. As mentioned, Lactium is a tiny molecule, and food will mask its effects. The second time, I took it without food, and in exactly three and a half weeks, I finally felt a shift in my stress levels. That is when I knew I had optimized my genes! And believe me, it was a very, very nice feeling.

Finally, as mentioned above, if at any point you decide, in conjunction with your healthcare practitioner, to wean your child off of medication, think about suggestions in this book for lifestyle or supplements that could support your child through the process.

For example, if dopamine production or regulation is of concern, you would likely want to increase your child's tyrosine intake so that they can produce dopamine more naturally. Consider a combination of tyrosine and herbs like Rhodiola or vitamins like folate. We often recommend a combination supplement called DopaPlus in the US and FocusPlus in Canada. This supplement can support the medication-to-no-medication transition for clients whose COMT gene supports its use. The ability to tailor support supplements is one of the many benefits of understanding your child's genetics.

TRAVELER ASSISTANCE

I (Brenda) am very grateful that the first complementary practitioner who helped me on my journey to wellness decades ago was so diligent in teaching me how to choose supplements. At the time, he was a formulator for several of the major Canadian supplement companies and was scrupulous in how he practiced his skills.

The training Alicia and I have taken as Registered Holistic Nutritionists has reinforced my learned-long-ago criteria.

When evaluating the quality of supplements, we suggest you consider the following criteria:

- **Third-party testing:** Look for supplements tested by independent organizations like NSF, USP, or ConsumerLab to verify purity and potency.

- **Clear labeling:** Ensure the label provides detailed information on ingredients, dosage, and potential allergens or additives.

- **No artificial additives:** Choose supplements free from artificial colors, flavors, and preservatives.

- **Bioavailability:** Select supplements with nutrients easily easily absorbed and assimilated by the body (e.g., chelated minerals attached to an amino acid, such as magnesium glycinate).

- **Transparency:** Check for clear sourcing information and reputable manufacturing practices (e.g., Good Manufacturing Practices [GMP] certified facilities).

- **Company reputation:** Look for brands with good reviews, longevity in the market, and a focus on quality control.

REST STOP

It's time for parents to take a break and digest information! Take 10 minutes of calm to Rest with the following questions:

1. **Examine your beliefs about medical treatments:** What are your personal beliefs or concerns about using medications or alternative treatments for ADHD? How have your past experiences or societal influences shaped these perspectives, and could these beliefs influence your

decision-making for your child?

2. **Reflect on your openness to alternatives:** How open are you to exploring alternative therapies alongside traditional medical treatments or vice versa for your child's ADHD? Are any internal hesitations or fears holding you back from trying new approaches?

Next, Stop for 10 minutes of quiet (sitting or slowly walking). Keep your mind as clear and open as possible, and just listen. Jot down or tell Siri to "make a note" of any responses that may arise. Because you've taken time to ponder calmly and quietly, these responses will most likely be less off-the-cuff and from a deeper level. They can give you clues as to the reasons behind your answers! Those clues, in turn, will reveal potential problematic thinking and can provide great direction on moving forward with the recommendations in this chapter that would be the easiest to implement or fit best for your family!

ROADWORK

Medication or Supplement Monitoring Journal

Materials:

- Notebook or digital device, pen

Directions:

1. **Daily Log:** Record the medication or supplement taken, dosage, and time of day.

2. **Observations:** Note any changes in behavior, focus, appetite, and sleep.

3. **Side Effects:** List any side effects noticed, their severity, and duration.

4. **Weekly Review:** Review the journal with your child's healthcare provider to adjust the treatment plan as needed.

This journal can provide clues to help ensure that your child's medication and supplements are working effectively and safely. It can also provide a clear record to discuss with your healthcare provider.

As Dr. Maté mentions in his book *Scattered Minds: "Consider the long-term implications of medication use, not just its short-term benefits."* Dr. Mate continued, and we fully agree, that *"Medications should never be the only treatment, or even the first treatment."*

SOUVENIR

This Step's souvenir is to suggest that you work with your healthcare team to develop a list of supplements that make sense for your child's situation based on the information you've gleaned from your research and the information we've provided on supplements that support various body systems.

Then, purchase high-quality supplements per this Step's Traveler Assistance. Brands that we like and have found particularly helpful are Pure Encapsulations, Designs for Health, Signature Supplements (which is Canada-based and only available through a practitioner but can be shipped to the US), and Genestra (specifically, their quality line of HMF probiotics).

Chapter 14

Conclusion

Parenting a child with ADHD (whether or not they have had an official diagnosis) is a bit like Mark's and my (Brenda's) 25th wedding anniversary trip to Greece, where we navigated many a steep and winding road, signs in a language my husband hadn't studied since we were first married, multiple lane highways where drivers paid little attention to the lines, and numerous unexpected twists and turns. And as that trip did, despite many glitches, we hope it turns out well for your child and your relationship!

It's a journey that demands patience, creativity, and a whole lot of compassion. But here's the empowering truth: the more pieces of the DNA mosaic you can decipher, understand their impact, and then adjust the environment in a way that fosters optimal expression of those genes, the easier it becomes to be aware of potentially challenging situations before they happen, and put practices in place to manage challenging thinking or behaviors before they escalate. This understanding gives you a sense of control and confidence in navigating your unique family dynamics.

Throughout these pages, we've explored a holistic approach to managing ADHD, integrating scientific research with practical, everyday strategies. We've delved into the seven Core **ELEVATE** Steps—**E-Eat for Energy, L-Love to Move, E-Enjoy Sleep, V-Value Detox, A-Access Calm, T-Target Inflammation, and E-Engage Repair**—each designed to optimize the functions of genes in that category that potentially impact ADHD symptoms. Rather than being another parenting manual for children with ADHD, it's a comprehensive guide that respects your child's genetic individuality while offering options for helping your child best manage situations that are a mismatch for their unique and wonderfully made brain functioning.

By understanding how genetics and the environment interact, you're equipped with powerful knowledge and actionable strategies to make informed decisions that support your child's well-being. Whether it's tweaking their diet to enhance focus and minimize blood sugar spikes, ensuring they get quality sleep, incorporating mindfulness practices to calm their minds, or providing supplements that support nutritional deficiencies and neurotransmitter functioning, you have a toolkit of unique and effective strategies.

We've also emphasized the importance of viewing ADHD through a lens of potential and opportunity. ADHD isn't a deficit; it's a difference that comes with its own set of strengths. By holding that perspective, you can help your child harness their creativity, enthusiasm, and out-of-the-box thinking to thrive in a world that often demands conformity.

Now, it's your turn to apply what you've learned to your family's daily life. Remember, without action, there are no results. But at the same time, this journey isn't about perfection; it's about progress. Celebrate the small victories—your child's and your own—and please practice the liberal use of kindness and compassion when things don't go as planned.

Parenting a child with ADHD is an ongoing process that requires adaptability, patience, emotional growth, and an open heart. Approach each day with hope, knowing you're making a difference in your child's life.

And, please, don't go through this journey alone. Take the time and effort to share your stories—successes and challenges. Engage with other parents navigating similar paths. Reach out to us with questions or for more information on our online Epigenetic Approach to Parenting Children with ADHD courses (info@www.inbalancelm.com)!

We can all learn from each other by fostering a community of mutual support.

As I (Alicia) reflected on my life's journey while writing this book, both as an entrepreneur in health and wellness and as a mother, I recognized that some of the toughest lessons come from experiences we'd rather forget. There was a time when my struggles with metabolizing dopamine and managing stress would lead to anger I couldn't contain. In those moments, I saw hurt in the eyes of my children, and a deep sorrow filled my heart, knowing I had unintentionally caused them pain.

I once believed I inherited these challenges, and the guilt was overwhelming. But learning about epigenetics was like finding a lost piece of the puzzle. It's more than just science; it's personal. It has allowed me to validate my struggles by understanding the genetic roadmap that makes me who I am. This is not an excuse but an explanation, and it has brought me a profound sense of acceptance. With this knowledge, I learned to embrace my uniqueness, forgive my past as a mother, and step into my professional role with renewed confidence and self-compassion.

Sharing this isn't easy, but if it can inspire even one parent grappling with ADHD solutions to look at their challenges through the lens of epigenetics and feel hopeful and valued, then the challenges I had in the past would have been worth it. Embrace the journey of discovery—our weaknesses can become our greatest strengths.

A Celebratory We Did It Review!

Wow, we've reached the end of our journey together through the *Epigenetic Roadmap for Parenting Children with ADHD!* We hope you've found the tools and insights in this book helpful and that they have sparked some exciting changes in how you parent your child with ADHD and how your child honors their neurodiversity and manages situational mismatches.

Now, we have a small favor to ask. If this book helped you see ADHD in a new light or has changed how your household responds to your child with ADHD, please leave a review on Amazon. Your feedback not only helps us serve you better but also guides others who are searching for the same answers.

Leaving a review is easy. Simply head to your Amazon account, click purchases, and then click our book and leave a review or visit this link and share your thoughts!(https://geni.us/ReviewChildrenwithADHD)

That's it, except to say your support in this way is much appreciated!

Finally, before we conclude, we want to express our sincere gratitude for your commitment to understanding and supporting your child with ADHD. We hope you are already starting to practice many of the tips, techniques, and hands-on strategies we have suggested throughout these pages.

The bottom line is that your dedication and love are the cornerstones of your child's success. You play a vital role in shaping your child's future and believe it or not, your efforts will not go unnoticed.

Recently, I (Brenda) received a text from Rachel. It was a screenshot of one of her "memories on Facebook" from 14 years ago, when she was 16 or 17. In response to Facebook's universal "What's on your mind?" question, her post from that day said, "... is way beyond ready to move out."

Along with Rachel's screenshot, when she texted me, she commented, "Hmmm ... sounds like a prime Lyme disease reaction" (and, I'd add, an undiagnosed ADHD reaction). But in true testimony to the power of positive family dynamics and building lasting connections, her text continued, "Glad you helped me get through it!"

I'll reiterate. Some days, when ADHD and Lyme Disease conspired to combust Rachel and our whole household ... I wondered if there was going to be light at the end of the tunnel. Today, our thriving, loving, and solid relationship is testimony to the essential role of dedication and unconditional love!

Along with cheering you on in your commitment to your child's well-being, we have also aimed to give you an additional foundational piece: support in optimizing your child's (and your) genetic blueprint.

We hope that these guidelines will give you hope that there are alternatives or complementary support to the many different ADHD medications available and that we've been able to put you back in the driver's seat as the person responsible for family wellness.

We also hope that by the time your child is ready to move out of your household, they will, like our children, pack with them the healthy lifestyle habits you've helped instill in them.

As co-authors, we are honored to have shared this journey with you. Thank you for allowing us to be part of it.

Chapter 15

Glossary of Terms

Here's a glossary of terms from the book that might be unfamiliar.

ADHD (Attention-Deficit/Hyperactivity Disorder): A neurodevelopmental condition characterized by challenges with attention, impulsivity, and hyperactivity. ADHD is not a deficit but a difference in how the brain processes information and regulates emotions. It is often linked to unique strengths like creativity and adaptability.

Adiponectin: A hormone produced by fat cells that regulates insulin sensitivity and the metabolism and storage of fats and reduces inflammation.

Adrenal Glands: Glands that sit above each kidney and produce hormone messengers, including cortisol.

Allele: A variant form of a gene. As humans have two copies of each gene, we have two alleles, one inherited from each parent.

Amino Acid: The building blocks of proteins in the body. Certain amino acids, like tyrosine, play a critical role in producing neurotransmitters such as dopamine, which are essential for focus, motivation, and emotional regulation.

Autonomic Nervous System: The part of the nervous system that is not under conscious or voluntary control. It is responsible for functions such as blood pressure, heart rate, and sweating, among others.

Base Pair: The "rungs" of the DNA double-helix molecules comprise bonded pairs of the nucleic acids guanine (G), cytosine (C), adenine (A), and thymine (T).

Behavioral Therapy: A form of therapy that helps individuals understand how thoughts, feelings, and behaviors are interconnected.

CBT (Cognitive Behavioral Therapy): A type of therapy that helps children and adults identify unhelpful thought patterns and develop healthier ways of thinking and responding to challenges. It's often used to address anxiety, intrusive thoughts, and impulsivity in ADHD.

Carbohydrates: A food type containing chains of sugar molecules.

Central Nervous System: The main part of the nervous system which includes the spinal cord and brain.

Chromosome: The structure within cells into which DNA is organized.

Complex Carbohydrates: Carbohydrate sources that are not easily broken down and absorbed as simple sugars, which include vegetables, fruit, and legumes.

Co-Regulation: A process where a caregiver helps a child calm down and regulate their emotions by offering comfort, modeling calm behavior, and using supportive strategies. Co-regulation is a foundational step toward helping children learn to self-regulate.

Cortisol: The body's primary stress hormone produced by the adrenal glands.

DNA: Deoxyribonucleic acid is the molecule within cells that makes up chromosomes. It carries your individual genetic information.

Dominant: Term applied to an allele if it is expressed in a person who has only one of that allele. It overpowers a recessive allele.

Dopamine: A neurotransmitter (chemical messenger in the brain) responsible for reward, motivation, focus, and regulating emotional responses. Many ADHD treatments focus on balancing dopamine levels to improve attention and reduce impulsivity.

DRD2: D2 dopamine receptor in the brain.

Epigenetics: The study of how lifestyle and environmental factors, such as diet, sleep, movement, and stress, influence gene expression—turning genes "on" or "off"—without changing the genetic code itself.

Executive Functioning: A set of cognitive skills that help with planning, organizing, time management, self-control, and decision-making. Children with ADHD often struggle with executive functioning, leading to difficulties in managing daily tasks.

Fats: Macronutrients made up of fatty acids, used by the body for energy, cell structure, and producing essential compounds like hormones.

GABA (Gaba-aminobutyric acid): A neurotransmitter involved in the reward system.

Gene: A specific section of DNA responsible for coding for a protein.

Gene Expression: The process by which a gene's information is used to create proteins or other molecules that affect how the body works. For example, depending on environmental or lifestyle factors, a gene linked to dopamine production may be expressed differently.

Genome: The entire human DNA set, including all genes.

Genotype: The unique set of genetic instructions inherited from your child's biological parents. Variations in specific genes can influence how your child's brain processes dopamine, serotonin, and other chemicals that impact ADHD-related traits.

Heterozygous: A genetic term meaning that a person has inherited two different versions (alleles) of a gene—one from each biological parent. For example, in a heterozygous variant, only one allele may affect dopamine signaling.

HIIT (high-intensity interval training): An exercise training that alternates vigorous bouts of activity, such as sprinting, with lower-intensity recovery periods.

Homozygous Normal: A term used to describe a person who has inherited two "typical" or common versions of a gene from both biological parents. This means the gene likely functions as expected.

Homozygous Variant: Describes someone who has inherited two altered versions of a gene, one from each parent. This can influence how the body processes neurotransmitters or responds to stress, impacting ADHD traits.

HPA Axis: An acronym for the hypothalamic-pituitary-adrenal axis or stress pathway connecting the brain with the adrenal glands.

Leptin: A hormone produced by fat cells that decreases appetite and increases energy expenditure.

Lipid: Fat or fatty substances, including fatty acids, oils, waxes, and steroid hormones.

Metabolism: The overall term for the ongoing chemical processes in the body that burn food and produce energy.

Methylation: An inheritable chemical modification of DNA that affects gene expression.

Monogenic: A trait that is controlled by one gene.

Neurodivergence: A term that recognizes and celebrates differences in how brains function and process information, such as ADHD, autism, and dyslexia. These differences are not deficits but unique ways of thinking, feeling, and experiencing the world.

Neurotransmitters: Chemicals in the brain, like dopamine and serotonin, that transmit signals between neurons (nerve cells). Neurotransmitter imbalances can influence mood, focus, and energy levels, which are often areas of concern for children with ADHD.

Non-Stimulant Medications: Medications used to manage ADHD symptoms that do not increase dopamine levels in the brain. These medications often focus on regulating norepinephrine and may be a better fit for children who experience side effects from stimulant medications.

Normal Allele: Typically the original or baseline allele and usually not associated with increased risk. It is also called ancestral allele, standard allele, wild allele, or reference allele.

Nucleotide Base: One of the basic structural building blocks of DNA or RNA. They are adenine (A), guanine (G), cytosine (C), and thymine (T) (uracil (U) in RNA).

Nutrigenomics: The study of interactions between diet/nutrition and gene expression.

Nutritional Supplementation: The use of vitamins, minerals, and herbs for preventive and therapeutic purposes.

Phenotype: The human effect of our gene coding (**Genotype**). This can be anything from appearance, such as eye color, to functions such as metabolism and disease risk.

Polygenic: A trait that is influenced by a number of genes.

Positive Reinforcement: A behavioral strategy that rewards desired actions to encourage their recurrence.

Prefrontal Cortex: The front part of the brain responsible for executive functioning, decision-making, and emotional regulation. In children with ADHD, the prefrontal cortex often develops or functions at a different pace, contributing to challenges in these areas.

Protein: Macromolecule containing chains of amino acids used primarily to rebuild the body and produce many vital molecules such as enzymes and hormones.

Receptors: Membrane-bound molecules with specific sites for other molecules, such as hormones and neurotransmitters, to bind into.

Recessive: A term applied to an allele if it is only expressed in a person who has two copies of that allele. It is overpowered by a dominant allele.

Regulation (Emotional or Self-Regulation): The ability to manage emotions, behavior, and responses to external stimuli. Children with ADHD often need support in learning how to self-regulate, especially during moments of stress or frustration.

Reward System: The brain's mechanism for processing rewards and motivation. It is heavily influenced by dopamine. In ADHD, this system often seeks immediate gratification, which can make delayed rewards or long-term tasks feel less appealing.

rs Number: A reference number for a specific SNP (**Single Nucleotide Polymorphism**). It stands for Reference SNP cluster ID.

Serotonin: A chemical messenger that is important in the control of mood and craving.

Simple Carbohydrate: A simple form of sugar such as glucose, lactose, and fructose, which is rapidly absorbed into the bloodstream. Simple carbohydrates include foods such as bread, potatoes, corn, rice, fruit, and sweets.

Situational Mismatch: When a genetic predisposition for certain behaviors, traits, or responses does not align well with the current environment or situation. This mismatch can lead to challenges or maladaptive outcomes, even though the same genetic trait may have been advantageous in a different context or era. For example, characteristics such as impulsivity or hyperactivity, which may have been beneficial for survival in highly dynamic or risky environments, can present difficulties in modern settings, prioritizing structure and prolonged focus.

SNP (Single Nucleotide Polymorphism): A small variation in a gene that can affect how it functions. For example, certain SNPs influence dopamine production or how the body manages stress, which can play a role in ADHD traits.

Stimulant Medications: Medications that increase levels of dopamine and norepinephrine in the brain, helping improve focus, attention, and impulse control. In the medical world, these are often the first line of treatment for ADHD.

Stress Cycle: The body's natural process for responding to and recovering from stress. Completing the stress cycle through physical activity, breathing exercises, or creative outlets helps prevent burnout and improves emotional well-being.

Trait: A particular characteristic of an individual that results from certain genetic coding, for example, eye color.

Tyrosine: An amino acid that serves as a precursor to dopamine production. Including tyrosine-rich foods (e.g., almonds, chicken, avocado) or supplements can help support focus and motivation in children with ADHD.

Variant Allele: Typically, the abnormal or risk allele for a SNP. It is also called risk allele, derived allele, mutant allele, or atypical allele.

Chapter 16

Appendix 1 - SNPs

H ere is a listing of the primary SNPs covered in this book. Again, a SNP is a small variation in a gene that can affect its function. Specific SNPs influence dopamine production or how the body manages stress, which can play a role in ADHD traits.

If you have your child's DNA tested, you can check for SNP coding to see if the SNPs are normal, heterozygous, or variant. The coding will indicate which of the book's Core Steps are most important to consider as starting points for honoring your child's neurodivergence and helping them better manage situational mismatches.

APPENDIX 1 - SNPS

METABOLIC

SNP	CODING	NORMAL	HETEROZYGOUS	VARIANT
MCR4	rs17782313	TT	TC	CC
ADIPOQ	rs17366568	GG	GA	AA
ADRB2	rs1042714	CC	CG	GG
** PPARG	rs1801282	CC	CG	GG

MACROS: PROTEIN, FAT

FTO	rs9939609	TT	TA	AA

MACROS: CARBOHYDRATES

GIPR	rs2287019	CC	CT	TT
TCF7L2	rs7903146	CC	CT	TT
IRS1	rs2943641	TT	TC	CC

MACROS: FATS

FABP2	rs142649876	GG	GA	AA
APOA2	rs5082	AA	AG	GG

MOVE

ACTN3	rs1815739	CC	CT	TT
ADRB2	rs1042713	GG	GA	AA
ACE	rs4343	GG	GA	AA

SLEEP

CLOCK	rs1801260	AA	AG	GG
CRY1	rs8192440	AA	AG	GG

DETOXIFICATION - PHASE 1

CYP1A2	rs762551	AA	AC	CC
CYP3A4	rs2740574	CC	CT	TT

NOTE: ** Variant has beneficial properties

APPENDIX 1 - SNPS

DETOXIFICATION - PHASE 2

SNP	CODING	NORMAL	HETEROZYGOUS	VARIANT
SOD2	rs4880	AA	AG	GG
GSTP1	rs1695	AA	AG	GG
NQO1	rs1800566	GG	GA	AA

CALM

COMT	rs4680	GG	GA	AA
DRD2	rs6277	AA	AG	GG
DAT1	rs463379	CC	CG	GG
TPH2	rs4570625	GG	GT	TT
** MAOA	rs77905	GG	GA	AA
FKBP5	rs3800373	CC	CA	AA
CRHR1	rs242939	TT	TC	CC
GAD1	rs2241165	CC	CT	TT

INFLAMMATION

IL6	rs1800795	CC	CG	GG
TNFa	rs1800629	GG	GA	AA

REPAIR

SIRT6	rs352493	TT	TC	CC
** FOXO3	rs2802292	TT	TG	GG
BDNF	rs6265	CC	CT	CC

OTHER

MTHFR	rs1801131	TT	TG	GG
FUT2	rs602662	GG	GA	AA

NOTE: ** Variant has beneficial properties

Chapter 17

Appendix 2 – Diagnosing ADHD

D iagnosing ADHD involves more than noticing that your child has trouble sitting still or paying attention. The DSM-5 (Diagnostic and Statistical Manual of Mental Disorders, Fifth Edition) outlines the criteria. Children up to age 16 must exhibit at least six inattention and/or hyperactivity-impulsivity symptoms, while adolescents (17+) and adults must have five or more.

1. Inattention:

- Often fails to pay attention to details or makes careless mistakes.

- Difficulty sustaining attention in tasks or play.

- Does not seem to listen when spoken to directly.

- Often does not follow through on instructions or fails to finish tasks.

- Has difficulty organizing tasks and activities.

- Avoids or dislikes tasks that require sustained mental effort.

- Often loses items needed for tasks or activities.

- Easily distracted by extraneous stimuli.

- Frequently forgetful in daily activities.

2. Hyperactivity and Impulsivity:
   - Often fidgets with hands or feet or squirms in their seat.

   - Leaves seat in situations where remaining seated is expected.

   - Runs or climbs in inappropriate situations (in adults, may feel restless).

   - Unable to play or engage in activities quietly.

   - Often "on the go" or acts as if "driven by a motor."

   - Talks excessively.

   - Blurts out answers before questions have been completed.

   - Difficulty waiting their turn.

   - Interrupts or intrudes on others' conversations or games.

These symptoms must persist for at least six months, be inappropriate for the individual's developmental level, and be present in two or more settings, such as home and school, or for teens, a part-time job. The symptoms must also interfere with or reduce the quality of social or academic functioning. These criteria ensure a comprehensive diagnosis considering the broader impact on the child's life.

Various tools and tests assess ADHD. Rating scales like the Conners' Rating Scale and the Vanderbilt ADHD Diagnostic Parent Rating Scale are widely recognized for their validity in measuring symptoms across multiple settings. These scales involve questionnaires completed by parents, teachers, and sometimes the child, providing subjective information from various sources.

Behavioral assessments, like the Test of Variables of Attention (TOVA), offer more objective data by measuring attention and impulsivity. The TOVA uses computerized tasks to assess a child's ability to sustain attention and control impulses. While valuable, these tools are just one part of the diagnostic process.

Diagnosing ADHD can be challenging, particularly for individuals with milder symptoms or those who don't fit the stereotypical profile. A quietly inattentive child, for example, may not be seen as someone needing assessment, especially if they aren't disruptive. Girls are often underdiagnosed, as their symptoms—potentially daydreaming or overthinking—differ from the overt hyperactivity typically seen in boys. ADHD also shares symptoms with other conditions, like anxiety, depression, and learning disabilities, making thorough assessment crucial to avoid misdiagnosis and inappropriate treatment.

Chapter 18

Appendix 3 – Supplements

Per our reasoning in the book about quality and effectiveness, we primarily recommend three supplement brands: Pure Encapsulations (unless otherwise indicated, the following supplements are made by Pure Encapsulations), Signature Supplements (SS), and Genestra's HMF line for probiotics. Should you need help accessing these brands, don't hesitate to contact us at info@inbalancelm.co. We can arrange dropshipping to most addresses in North America.

APPENDIX 3 - ADHD SUPPLEMENTS

For DNA

	PURPOSE	SUPPORTS SNPS	DOSING
Focus Plus (Can) Dopa Plus (US) or L-Tyrosine	Provides Tyrosine and other supplements to promote dopamine production	COMT DRD2	1 cap twice a day for 8 weeks. Empty stomach. Then 1 a day for maintenance.
EFA Caps or Liquid (Omega 3s)	Support brain health and inflammation	IL6 BDNF	1 cap or 1 tsp once a day. With food.
Sereniten Plus or Stress Reset (SS)	Stress management and reduction.	Stress genes like FKBP5	1 cap twice a day, one in the morning, one 1.5 hrs before bedtime. Empty stomach.
NAC (N-Acetyl Cysteine)	Supports phase 2 liver detoxification and reduces inflammation	SOD2, GSTP1, NQO1 IL6, TNFa	1 cap twice a day 4 to 12 weeks, depending on genes Then 1 per day. Empty stomach.
Glutathione (Liposomal or S-Acetyl)	Supports phase 2 liver detoxification and reduces inflammation	SOD2, GSTP1, NQO1 IL6, TNFa	1 cap twice a day 4 to 12 weeks, depending on genes. Then 1 per day. Empty stomach.
DIM or DIM Detox (depending on CYP1A2 gene)	Supports phase 1 liver detoxification.	CYP1A2 CYP3A4	1 cap twice a day for 4 weeks, then 1 a day. Empty stomach.
Resveratrol	Antioxidant	IL6 BDNF SIRT6	1 cap twice a day for 8 weeks, then 1 a day. Empty stomach.

APPENDIX 3 - ADHD SUPPLEMENTS

For DNA

	PURPOSE	SUPPORTS SNPS	DOSING
Astaxanthin	Antioxidant	SOD2 FOXO3	1 cap twice a day for 8 weeks, then 1 a day. Empty stomach.
Neural Repair (SS): Contains Resveratrol, Astaxanthin & SOD2	Antioxidant	IL6, BDNF, SIRT6, SOD2, FOXO3	1 cap twice a day for 8 weeks, then 1 a day. Empty stomach.
Digestive Enzymes Ultra or GI Soothe (SS)	Digestive support	MC4R, ADIPOQ, FTO, GC	Take one cap when bloated or uncomfortable. GI Soothe supports mucous formation.
Melatonin	Promotes sleep	CLOCK CRY1	1 cap 1.5 hrs before bedtime.
Melatonin SR	Promotes sleep through the night	CLOCK CRY1	1 cap 1.5 hrs before bedtime.
Best Rest	Promotes sleep	CLOCK CRY1	1 cap 1.5 hrs before bedtime.
Magnesium Glycinate and Zinc Glycinate	Magnesium: Promotes relaxation Zinc: supports many cell functions	Magnesium: CLOCK CRY1 Zinc: SLC30A8	Magnesium: 1 cap or tsp 1.5 hrs before bedtime. Zinc: 1 tsp with a meal.

Chapter 19

Appendix 4 - Quick Wellness Steps

Wellness Steps for "Those" Days (AKA Cost-effective Strategies for Busy Days)

Parenting a child with ADHD is a demanding journey, and we know time, energy, and financial resources can often feel in short supply. Even if you haven't had your child's DNA tested or mapped out every piece of genetic data, there are straightforward, cost-effective steps you can take to support their overall wellness.

These small, manageable actions can have a meaningful impact, helping balance behaviors, improve focus, and foster a sense of calm for your child and your household. This appendix is designed for those moments when you need small, practical, easy-to-implement strategies that still make a big difference.

Core Step – Eat

Overview

This step focuses on the impact of food and nutrition on managing ADHD symptoms. From macronutrient balance to the importance of micronutrients and personalized nutrition, it offers actionable insights for parents.

Quick Steps for Wellness

1. **Breakfast Boost:** Start the day with a balanced breakfast, including protein (e.g., eggs), healthy fats (e.g., avocado), and fiber-rich carbs (e.g., whole-grain toast). This will stabilize blood sugar and support focus

throughout the morning.

2. **Veggie Variety Rule:** Aim for three colors of vegetables at every meal to encourage a nutrient-dense diet and improve gut health. This means you even start your day with veggies!

3. **Involve Your Child in Meal Prep:** Let your child help with grocery shopping or meal preparation to increase their willingness to try new foods and promote healthy eating habits.

Why This Works

Balanced meals provide the building blocks for neurotransmitters like dopamine and serotonin, which are crucial for attention and mood regulation. Engaging your child in food choices encourages a positive relationship with nutrition, reduces resistance, and fosters long-term healthy habits.

Core Step – Move

Overview

This step emphasizes the importance of movement in managing ADHD symptoms. Regular physical activity can regulate brain chemicals like dopamine and norepinephrine, fostering better focus, emotional regulation, overall well-being, and other lifestyle factors like sleep.

Quick Steps for Wellness

1. **Movement Breaks Between Tasks:** Encourage short bursts of activity—jumping jacks, skipping, or a quick dance break—between homework or chores to reset focus and boost energy.

2. **Family Movement Challenges:** Organize fun challenges, such as who can do the most squats, jumps, or steps in a day. Track progress on a family chart to build motivation.

3. **Encourage Nature Play:** Spend time in nature through hiking, climbing, or even backyard scavenger hunts. Being outdoors enhances movement and reduces stress.

Why This Works

Incorporating movement into daily life enhances dopamine and norepineph-rine levels, promotes teamwork and social bonding, and fosters joy in staying active. These steps balance structured activity with playful, spontaneous move-ment, making incorporating it into your family's routine easier.

Core Step – Sleep

Overview

This step focuses on improving your child's sleep quality and quantity by addressing genetic, behavioral, and environmental factors. Good sleep is foun-dational for managing ADHD symptoms and supporting overall brain health.

Quick Steps for Wellness

1. **Morning Light Exposure:** Take your child outside for 10–30 minutes of morning sunlight or use a SAD light if you live in locations with low light levels. This helps reset their circadian rhythm and energizes them for the day.

2. **Create a Wind-Down Zone:** Dedicate a specific area for quiet evening activities, like coloring, puzzles, or listening to audiobooks or binaural beats. Avoid stimulating tasks to help your child transition to sleep.

3. **Personalize the Sleep Space:** Invest in blackout curtains and a white noise machine to create a dark, quiet, and cool environment. Test what works best for your child's preferences.

Why This Works

These steps address both biological and environmental factors affecting sleep. Morning light exposure regulates circadian rhythms, wind-down activities ease the transition to bedtime, and a well-optimized sleep environment ensures a deeper, more restorative sleep cycle.

Core Step – Detox

Overview

This step focuses on supporting your child's natural detoxification processes to reduce the burden of environmental toxins, which can exacerbate ADHD symptoms. Simple changes in diet, daily routines, and household products can help create a cleaner, healthier environment and improve your child's overall well-being.

Quick Steps for Wellness

1. **Hydrate Often:** Encourage your child to drink plenty of water daily. Proper hydration supports kidney function and toxin elimination. Add a slice of lemon or a few berries to the water for flavor if needed.

2. **Use Epsom Salt Baths:** Add one to two cups of Epsom salts to a warm bath and let your child soak for 20–30 minutes. The magnesium helps relax muscles, calm the nervous system, and promote toxin release.

3. **Incorporate Daily Movement:** Encourage activities like walking, biking, or playing outdoors. Physical activity helps stimulate lymphatic flow, aiding in removing waste products from the body.

Why This Works

These steps enhance your child's detoxification pathways by supporting key elimination organs like the kidneys, skin, and lymphatic system. Hydration and movement assist in flushing toxins, while Epsom salt baths offer a relaxing and accessible way to support detoxification and calmness.

Core Step – Calm

Overview

This step focuses on helping your child manage stress and achieve a sense of calm by addressing neurotransmitter regulation, establishing supportive routines, and fostering emotional resilience. These strategies provide immediate relief and lay the foundation for long-term well-being.

Quick Steps for Wellness

1. **Create a Morning Routine with Predictable Visuals:** Outline your child's morning routine using a visual schedule with images or checklists. This minimizes decision-making stress and creates a calming, predictable start to the day.

2. **Encourage Movement Breaks:** Implement short physical activity

breaks, such as jumping jacks, stretches, or a quick game of tag. These release pent-up energy, provide a dopamine boost and improve focus.

3. **Practice Mindful Breathing Together:** Teach your child belly breathing to engage the parasympathetic nervous system. Inhale deeply for 4 seconds, hold for 2, and exhale for 6 seconds. Practice together to model calmness.

Why This Works

These steps target key challenges children with ADHD face in maintaining emotional regulation and calmness. Routines and visual tools reduce cognitive load and anxiety, while mindfulness activities and movement breaks help the nervous system reset and manage energy levels. These small, consistent practices can create significant improvements in daily interactions.

Core Step – Inflammation

Overview

Inflammation is the body's natural response to injury or stress, but chronic inflammation can exacerbate ADHD symptoms and disrupt overall health. By reducing inflammatory triggers and supporting anti-inflammatory practices, you can help create a calmer, more balanced environment for your child.

Quick Steps for Wellness

1. **Hydrate with Purpose**: Encourage your child to drink water infused with a squeeze of lemon or a few cucumber slices. This adds a mild anti-inflammatory boost while ensuring proper hydration.

2. **Note Any Connection Between Food Intake and Gut Inflammation**. Replace any inflammation-triggering food with non-inflammatory whole food. Try new flavors, textures, and colored veggies.

3. **Snack Swap**: Replace sugary or processed snacks with anti-inflammatory options like fresh berries, almonds, or walnuts. These nutrient-dense foods can help combat inflammation and stabilize mood.

Why This Works

These steps are easy to implement and target inflammation from multiple angles—diet, hydration, and relaxation. Together, they can help reduce stress and inflammation, creating a supportive environment for managing ADHD symptoms.

Core Step – Repair

Overview

This step focuses on supporting your child's DNA repair processes, which play a crucial role in managing ADHD symptoms and promoting overall brain health. Addressing oxidative stress and enhancing the body's natural repair mechanisms can help optimize your child's neurological functioning.

Quick Steps for Wellness

1. **Serve a Rainbow Plate:** Include five different-colored fruits and vegetables in your child's meals daily to boost antioxidant intake. Think of this as a "toolbox" full of protective tools for their DNA.

2. **Encourage Screen-Free Evenings:** To reduce oxidative stress and improve sleep quality, create a calming, screen-free hour before bed. Swap screens for quiet activities like reading or drawing.

3. **Promote Sleep Hygiene:** Ensure your child gets enough quality sleep, as deep sleep is essential for cellular repair and brain recovery.

Why This Works

These steps help mitigate oxidative stress, a significant disruptor of DNA repair, and foster the body's natural ability to heal and maintain itself. A colorful diet provides antioxidants, and quality sleep allows the body to reset and repair.

Supplemental Essential One – Behavioral and Educational Strategies

Overview

This chapter offers practical strategies for parents to help their children manage their ADHD-related behaviors, support learning, and foster positive relationships. It introduces behavioral interventions, collaboration with schools, technology use, social skills training, and tools for emotional regulation.

Quick Steps for Wellness

1. **Establish Positive Reinforcement:** Create a token system where your child earns points for tasks or good behavior, which can be redeemed for rewards like a family game night or extra playtime.

2. **Use Environmental Adjustments:** Organize clutter-free spaces and provide sensory aids (e.g., stress balls and weighted blankets) to reduce overstimulation and improve focus.

3. **Role-play Social Scenarios:** To improve confidence and social interactions, you can use a tennis ball game to practice conversational skills, such as making statements and asking questions.

Why This Works

These strategies address behavior through structured routines, emotional regulation techniques, and environmental adjustments. They empower children with ADHD to develop self-regulation, enhance focus, and build social connections. Parents also gain tools to create a supportive and consistent framework for their child's growth.

Supplemental Essentials Two – ADHD Family Dynamics

Overview

This chapter explores the unique challenges and opportunities that ADHD brings to family life. It provides strategies for balancing attention among siblings, fostering understanding and empathy, prioritizing parental self-care, resolving conflicts, and creating an ADHD-friendly home environment.

Quick Steps for Wellness

1. **Balance Attention:** Schedule one-on-one time with each child regularly, even briefly, to reassure them of their unique importance in the family.

2. **Model Self-Care:** Incorporate activities like mindful breathing or a weekly hobby into your routine to show your children the importance of mental and physical health.

3. **Complete the Stress Cycle:** Teach stress-reducing practices such as physical activity, mindful breathing, and creative outlets to help your child discharge pent-up energy and reset emotionally.

Why This Works

By creating an environment that values each family member's needs and provides tools for managing ADHD, you foster resilience, understanding, and harmony within the household. These practices also build essential life skills like self-regulation, empathy, and effective communication.

Supplemental Essentials Three – Medical and Alternative Treatments

Overview

Navigating ADHD treatments can feel overwhelming, but this chapter illuminates key strategies and options, including behavioral therapies, medications, and supplements. By understanding the interconnectedness of genetics, environmental influences, and personalized approaches, you can build a comprehensive, informed plan tailored to your child's needs.

Quick Steps for Wellness

1. **Behavioral Therapy as Part of Your Plan:** Explore behavioral modification, CBT, and social skills training as foundational interventions. These approaches can provide lasting tools for emotional regulation and improved behavior.

2. **Understand Medications:** Work with your healthcare provider to determine if ADHD medications might help your child. Monitor for side effects and personalize the plan based on genetics, environmental factors, and observed responses.

3. **Integrate Supplements:** Consider natural supplements, such as tyrosine, magnesium, omega-3s, and zinc, to support ADHD management. Use the Traveler Assistance tips to choose high-quality options.

4. **Complete the Picture:** Address stress, inflammation, and detoxification through the lifestyle recommendations in this book to complement medical or alternative treatments.

Why This Works

By combining therapies, treatments, and lifestyle changes with a focus on personalization, you can address ADHD's multifaceted nature. This approach supports symptom management and long-term emotional and physical health, empowering your child to thrive.

Chapter 20

Selected References and Resources

This book could not have been written without the hundreds of diligent researchers, practitioners, and writers that went before us. Here are some of our most valued references and resources.

EPIGENETICS AND GENERAL REFERENCES

- Amen, D. G. 1998. *Change your brain, change your life: The break-through program for conquering anxiety, depression, obsessiveness, lack of focus, anger, and memory problems.* Harmony Books.

- DNA Testing: www.dnaallure.com Kit: Ultimate Genomics.

- Greenblatt, J & Gottlieb, B. 2017. *Finally Focused.* Harmony Books.

- Greene, R. W. (2014). *The explosive child: A new approach for understanding and parenting easily frustrated, chronically inflexible children* (5th ed.). HarperCollins.

- Kendall-Reed P & Reed S. 2020. *Fix your Genes to Fit your Jeans.* Tell-Well, Canada.

- Lankerani A. 2024. *The Parenting Owner's Manual: The A to Zs of raising a happy, healthy family from experts around the world.*

- Lieberman, D. Z., & Long, M. E. (2018). *The molecule of more: How a single chemical in your brain drives love, sex, and creativity—and will determine the fate of the human race.* BenBella Books.

- Lynch B. 2018. *Dirty Genes.* Harper One.

- Mate,G. 2024. *Scattered Minds. The Origins and Healing of Attention Deficit Disorder.* Vintage Canada.

- Mate, G. *ADHD.* https://drgabormate.com/adhd/

- Melillo, R. 2015. *Disconnected Kids: The Groundbreaking Brain Balance Program for Children with Autism, ADHD, Dyslexia, and Other Neurological Disorders.* 3rd ed. Penguin Books.

- Murgia, M. 2017. *The chemical mind: CrashCourse psychology #3* [Video]. YouTube. https://www.youtube.com/watch?v=Wuy-PuH9ojCE

- Mukherjee S. 2017. *The Gene, An Intimate Story.* Penguin Random House, UK.

- Neale B.M. et al. 2010. Meta-analysis of genome-wide association studies of attention deficit/hyperactivity disorder. *J Am Acad Child Adolesc Psychiatry* 49(9): 884–897

- Neufeld G & Mate G. 2013. *Hold On to Your Kids. Why Parents Need to Matter More than Peers.* Vintage Canada.

- Tonti, S. 2013. *ADHD as a difference in cognition, not a disorder.* TEDxCMU. YouTube. https://www.youtube.com/watch?v=uU6o2_UFSEY

- Van der Kolk B. 2016. *The Body Keeps the Score.* Penguin Books.

- Wollenberg, B. 2024. *Metabolic Health Roadmap: Step-by-step epigenetic guide to revitalize energy levels, sharpen cognitive function, cultivate emotional wellbeing, and customize nutritional intake.*

UNDERSTANDING ADHD AND ITS FOUNDATIONS

- Centers for Disease Control and Prevention (CDC). 2020. Data and statistics about ADHD. Retrieved from https://www.cdc.gov

- Conners, C. K., Pitkanen, J., & Rzepa, S. R. 2011. Conners Comprehensive Behavior Rating Scales (CBRS). *MHS Assessments. https://storefront.mhs.com/collections/conners-cbrs*

- Cortese, S. 2012. The neurobiology and genetics of Attention-Deficit/Hyperactivity Disorder (ADHD): What every clinician should know. *European Journal of Paediatric Neurology* 16: 422-433.

- Greenberg, L. M., & Waldman, I. D. 1993. Developmental normative data on the Test of Variables of Attention (TOVA). *Journal of Child Psychology and Psychiatry 34*(6): 1019-1030.

- Hinshaw, S. P., & Scheffler, R. M. 2014. *The ADHD Explosion: Myths, Medication, Money, and Today's Push for Performance.* Oxford University Press.

- Polanczyk, G., de Lima, M. S., Horta, B. L., Biederman, J., & Rohde, L. A. 2007. The worldwide prevalence of ADHD: A systematic review and metaregression analysis. *American Journal of Psychiatry* 164(6): 942-948.

- Posner, J., Polanczyk, G. V., & Sonuga-Barke, E. 2020. Attention-deficit hyperactivity disorder. *The Lancet* 395(10222): 450-462.

- Rohr, R. 2024. *Richard Rohr's Daily Meditations.* Center for Action and Contemplation. Meditations@cac.org

- Rubia, K. 2018. Cognitive Neuroscience of Attention Deficit Hyperactivity Disorder (ADHD) and its Clinical Translation. *Frontiers in Human Neuroscience* 12: 100.

- Thapar, A., Cooper, M., Eyre, O., & Langley, K. 2012. What have we learnt about the causes of ADHD? *Journal of Child Psychology and Psychiatry* 54(1): 3-16.

ADHD LONGER TERM AND DIAGNOSIS

- Amen, D.G. 2013. *Healing ADD. The breakthrough program that allows you to see and heal the 7 types of ADD*. Berkley, NY

- American Psychiatric Association. (2013). *Diagnostic and statistical manual of mental disorders* (5th ed.). American Psychiatric Association.

- Arnsten, A. F. T. 2009. The Emerging Neurobiology of Attention Deficit Hyperactivity Disorder: The Key Role of the Prefrontal Association Cortex. *Journal of Pediatrics* 154(5): I-S43.

- Arnsten, A. F. T. 2009. Stress signalling pathways that impair prefrontal cortex structure and function. *Nature Reviews Neuroscience* 10(6): 410-422.

- Arnsten, A. F. T., & Rubia, K. 2012. Neurobiological Circuits Regulating Attention, Cognitive Control, Motivation, and Emotion: Disruptions in Neurodevelopmental Psychiatric Disorders. *Journal of the American Academy of Child & Adolescent Psychiatry* 51(4): 356-367.

- Bush, G., Valera, E. M., & Seidman, L. J. 2005. Functional Neuroimaging of Attention-Deficit/Hyperactivity Disorder: A Review and Suggested Future Directions. *Biological Psychiatry* 57(11): 1273-1284.

- CDC. Diagnosing ADHD. https://www.cdc.gov/adhd/diagnosis/index.html

- Cecil, C. and Nigg, J. *2022.* Epigenetics and ADHD: Reflections on Current Knowledge, Research Priorities and Translation Potential. *Mol. Diag. Ther.* 6(6):581–606.

- Cubillo, A., & Rubia, K. 2010. Structural and Functional Brain Imaging in Adult Attention-Deficit/Hyperactivity Disorder. *Expert Review of Neurotherapeutics*, 10(4): 603-620.

- Exceptional Individuals. https://exceptionalindividuals.com

- Felt BT, Biermann B, Christner JG, Kochhar P, Harrison RV. 2014. Diagnosis and management of ADHD in children. *Am Fam Physician* Oct 1;90(7):456-64.

- Huberman, A, ADHD, Drive and Motivation. https://www.huberm anlab.com/topics/adhd-drive-and-motivation

- Mayo Clinic. (n.d.). *ADHD: Diagnosis and treatment.* Mayo Foundation for Medical Education and Research. https://www.mayoclinic.or g/diseases-conditions/adhd/diagnosis-treatment/drc-20350895

- McEwen, B. S., & Morrison, J. H. 2013. The Brain on Stress: Vulnerability and Plasticity of the Prefrontal Cortex Over the Life Course. *Neuron* 79(1), 16-29.

- Neufeld Institute. (n.d.). *Resources.* https://neufeldinstitute.org/resou rces/

- Purper-Ouakil, D, Ramoz, N, Lepagnol-Bestel, A, Gorwood, P, & Simonneau M. 2011. Neurobiology of Attention Deficit/Hyperactivity Disorder. *Pediatric Research* 69(5): 69R-76R

- Seidman, L. J., Valera, E. M., & Makris, N. 2005. Structural brain imaging of attention-deficit/hyperactivity disorder. *Biological Psychiatry* 57(11): 1263-1272.

- Silk, T. J., Beare, R., Malpas, C., Adamson, C., Vilgis, V., Vance, A., & Bellgrove, M. A. 2016. Cortical Morphology in Attention Deficit/Hyperactivity Disorder: Contribution of Thickness and Surface Area to Volume. *Cortex* 82: 1-10.

EAT AND METABOLISM

- Bandura, A. 1977. *Social learning theory*. Prentice Hall.

- Cortese, S., Morcillo-Peñalver, C., Comoretto, R., Maffeis, C., & Zuddas, A. 2019. Association between serum adiponectin levels and attention-deficit/hyperactivity disorder (ADHD) in children and adolescents: A systematic review and meta-analysis. *Psychoneuroendocrinology* 103: 196-202.

- Eisenberg, N., Fabes, R. A., & Spinrad, T. L. 1992. Prosocial development in children. *Social Development 1*(2): 153–170.

- Hurd, N. M., & Zimmerman, M. A. 2010. Natural mentoring relationships among adolescent mothers: A study of resilience. *Journal of Research on Adolescence 20*(3): 789–809.

- Mota, NR. 2020. Cross-disorder genetic analyses implicate dopaminergic signaling as a biological link between Attention-Deficit/Hyperactivity Disorder and obesity measures. *Neuropsychopharmacology* 45: 1188-1195

- Faraone, S. V., Gizer, I. R., & Asherson, P. 2016. MC4R gene variants and their association with obesity and attention-deficit/hyperactivity disorder in children and adolescents. *Biological Psychiatry* 79(4): 434-440

- Shi, X. et al. 2021. Ghrelin modulates dopaminergic neuron formation and attention deficit hyperactivity disorder-like behaviors: From animals to human models. *Brain, Behavior, and Immunity* 94:327-337

- Abizaid, A. et.al. 2006. Ghrelin modulates the activity and synaptic input organization of midbrain dopamine neurons while promoting appetite. *J Clin Invest* 116 (12);3229-3239

- Howard, A. L., Robinson, M., Smith, G. J., Ambrosini, G. L., Piek, J. P., & Oddy, W. H. 2011. ADHD is associated with a "Western" dietary pattern in adolescents. *Journal of Attention Disorders* 15(5): 403-411.

- Kim, Y., & Chang, H. 2011. Correlation between attention deficit hyperactivity disorder and sugar consumption, quality of diet, and dietary behavior in school children. *Nutr Res Pract.* 5(3): 236-245.

- Olivardia, R. 2020. *ADHD and disordered eating: ADHD essentials podcast with Roberto Olivardia, Ph.D.* [Video]. YouTube. https://www.youtube.com/watch?v=rozTN2l3SLM

EAT AND MACRONUTRIENTS

- *Brain Food: 11 ADHD Diet, Nutrition, and Supplement Rules* https://www.additudemag.com/adhd-nutrition-health-food-rules/

- Ellyn Satter Institute. (n.d.). *Ellyn Satter Institute: For the love of eating.* https://www.ellynsatterinstitute.org/

- Melhorn, S. J., Askren, M. K., Chung, W. K., Kratz, M., & Ren, X. 2016. FTO genotype is associated with phenotypic variability of dopamine D2 receptor availability and cognitive function in healthy individuals. *Neuropsychopharmacology* 41(1): 102-110.

- Milte, C. M., Parletta, N., Buckley, J. D., Coates, A. M., Young, R. M., & Howe, P. R. 2012. Eicosapentaenoic and docosahexaenoic acids, cognition, and behavior in children with attention-deficit/hyperactivity disorder: A randomized controlled trial. *Nutrition* 28(6): 670-677.

- Shulman, J. 2003. *Winning the food fight.* Wiley.

SLEEP

- *ADHD and Sleep Problems: How Are They Related?* https://www.slee pfoundation.org/mental-health/adhd-and-sleep

- *ADHD IEP Goals: A Complete Guide and Goal Bank.* https://www.par allellearning.com/post/adhd-iep-goals-a-complete-guide-and-goal-bank

- Bass, J., & Takahashi, J. S. 2010. Circadian integration of metabolism and energetics. *Science 330*(6009): 1349-1354.

- Carpena, M. X., & Hutz, M. H. 2019. CLOCK Polymorphisms in Attention-Deficit/Hyperactivity Disorder (ADHD): Further Evidence Linking Sleep and Circadian Disturbances and ADHD. *Journal of Neural Transmission* 126(6): 711-719.

- Cortese, S., Faraone, S. V., Konofal, E., & Lecendreux, M. 2013. Sleep in children with attention-deficit/hyperactivity disorder: Meta-analysis of subjective and objective studies. *Journal of the American Academy of Child & Adolescent Psychiatry 52*(4): 383–396.

- Curtis, A. M., Bellet, M. M., Sassone-Corsi, P., & O'Neill, L. A. J. 2014. Circadian clock proteins and immunity. *Immunity 40*(2): 178-186.

- McClung, C. A. 2013. How might circadian rhythms control mood? Let me count the ways. *Biological Psychiatry 74*(4): 242-249.

- Sancar, A., Lindsey-Boltz, L. A., Kang, T. H., Reardon, J. T., Lee, J. H., & Ozturk, N. 2015. Circadian clock control of the cellular response to DNA damage. *FEBS Letters 589*(14): 2478-2484.

- Scheer, F. A., Hu, K., Evoniuk, H., Kelly, E. E., Malhotra, A., & Shea, S. A. 2009. Impact of the human circadian system, exercise, and their interaction on cardiovascular function. *Proceedings of the National Academy of Sciences 107*(20): 10691-10696.

DETOXIFICATION

- *10 Ways to Create a Non-Toxic Home - Mindful Family Medicine.* http s://mindfulfamilymedicine.com/10-ways-to-create-a-non-toxic-home/

- Curatolo, P., D'Agati, E., & Moavero, R. 2010. The neurobiological basis of ADHD: From neurotransmission to neuroanatomy. *Frontiers in Human Neuroscience* 4: 19.

- Hook-Sopko, A. 2021. The benefits of dry skin brushing + how to do it properly. *Green Child Magazine.* https://www.greenchild-magazine.com/benefits-dry-skin-brushing/

- Lee MJ, Chou M, Chou W, Huang c, Kuo H, Lee, S & Wang L. 2018. Heavy Metals' Effect on Susceptibility to Attention-Deficit/Hyperactivity Disorder: Implication of Lead, Cadmium, and Antimony. *Int J Environ Res Public Health* 15(6): 1221

CALM

- Banderet, L. E., & Lieberman, H. R. 1989. Tyrosine: Precursor of catecholamines and its role in cognitive function and stress. *Brain Research Bulletin* 22(5): 759-762.

- Birdsall, T. C. 1998. 5-Hydroxytryptophan: A clinically-effective serotonin precursor. *Alternative Medicine Review* 3(4): 271-280.

- Cerqueira, J. J., Mailliet, F., Almeida, O. F. X., Jay, T. M., & Sousa, N. 2007. The prefrontal cortex as a key target of the maladaptive response to stress. *The Journal of Neuroscience* 27(11): 2781-2787.

- Fernstrom, J. D., & Fernstrom, M. H. 2007. Tyrosine, phenylalanine, and catecholamine synthesis and function in the brain. *The Journal of Nutrition* 137(6 Suppl 1): 1539S-1547S

- Hasler, G. 2010. Pathophysiology of Depression: Do we have any solid evidence of interest to clinicians? *World Psychiatry* 9(3): 55-161.

- Low, K. 2022. *Why Children with ADHD Need Structure and Routines.* https://www.verywellmind.com/why-is-structure-important-for-kids-with-adhd-20747

- *Mindfulness for ADHD: Benefits and Activities for Kids.* https://hes-extraordinary.com/manage-adhd-mindfulness

- Shaw, K., Turner, J., & Del Mar, C. 2002. Tryptophan and 5-Hydroxytryptophan for depression. *Cochrane Database of Systematic Reviews* (1): CD003198.

- Ortner, N. 2018. *The Tapping Solution for Parents, Children & Teenagers.* Hay House Inc.

- Van Stralen, J.. 2016. Emotional dysregulation in children with attention-deficit/hyperactivity disorder. *Atten Defic Hyperact Disord.* 14;8(4):175–187.

- Zylowska, L. 2024. Meditation for the Bored and Restless: How to Practice Mindfulness with ADHD. *Additude.* https://www.additudemag.com/how-to-practice-mindfulness-adhd/

INFLAMMATION

- Anand, D., Colpo, G. D., Zeni, G., Zeni, C. P., & Teixeira, A. L. 2017. Attention-Deficit/Hyperactivity Disorder and Inflammation: What Does Current Knowledge Tell Us? A Systematic Review. *Frontiers in Psychiatry* 8: 228.

- Oades, R. D., Myint, A. M., Dauvermann, M. R., Schimmelmann, B. G., Schwarz, M. J., & Müller, N. 2010. Attention-deficit hyperactivity disorder (ADHD) and inflammation: The role of the cytokine interleukin-6 (IL-6). *Journal of Child Psychology and Psychiatry* 51(10): 1101-1108.

MOVE AND REPAIR

- CHADD. 2019. *What's up with athletes and ADHD?* Children and Adults with Attention-Deficit/Hyperactivity Disorder (CHADD). https://chadd.org/adhd-weekly/whats-up-with-athletes-and-adhd/

- Chojdak-Łukasiewicz, J., Konieczny, P., Ziemka-Nalecz, M., Strosznajder, J. B., & Zalewska, T. 2022. Role of Sirtuins in Physiology and Diseases of the Central Nervous System. *Biomedicines* 10(10): 2434.

- Doucleff, M. 2023. *'Anti-dopamine parenting' can curb a kid's craving for screens or sweets.* https://www.npr.org/sections/health-shots/2023/06/12/1180867083/tips-to-outsmart-dopamine-unhook-children-from-screens-sweet

- Halperin, J. M., Berwid, O. G., & O'Neill, S. 2014. Healthy body, healthy mind?: The effectiveness of physical activity to treat ADHD in children. *Child and Adolescent Psychiatric Clinics of North America* 23(4): 899-936.

- Polter, A. M., & Yang, S. 2018. FoxO Transcription Factors in the Brain: Regulation and Behavioral Manifestation. *Biological Psychiatry* 83(8): 759-769.

- Premier Sport Psychology. 2022. ADHD in athletes: What we see, what to do. *Premier Sport Psychology.* https://premiersportpsychology.com/2022/11/05/adhd-in-athletes-what-we-see-what-to-do/

BEHAVIORAL AND EDUCATIONAL STRATEGIES

- *ADHD IEP Goals: A Complete Guide and Goal Bank* https://www.parallellearning.com/post/adhd-iep-goals-a-complete-guide-and-goal-bank

- *Cognitive Behavioral Therapy for ADHD: How Can It Help?* https://psychcentral.com/adhd/cbt-for-adhd

- Greene, R. W. 2014. *The explosive child: A new approach for understand-*

ing and parenting easily frustrated, chronically inflexible children (5th ed.). HarperCollins.

ADHD FAMILY DYNAMICS - PARENTING RESOURCES

- Amen D.G. and Fay, C. 2001. *Raising Mentally Strong Kids.* Tyndale Refresh.

- Nagoski, E., & Nagoski, A. 2019. *Burnout: The secret to unlocking the stress cycle.* Ballantine Books.

- Nelsen, J. 2006. *Positive Discipline.* Ballantine Books.

- Pinsky, S. C. 2012. *Organizing solutions for people with ADHD: Tips and tools to help you take charge of your life and get organized.* Fair Winds Press.

MEDICAL AND ALTERNATIVE TREATMENTS

- ADDitude Editors. (n.d.). *ADHD burnout: Why it happens & how to avoid it. Attention Deficit Disorder Association.* https://add.org/adhd -burnout/

- *Behavioral Treatments for Kids With ADHD - Child Mind Institute* https://childmind.org/article/behavioral-treatments-kids-adhd/#:~:tex t=through%20parent%20training.-,School%20interventions,for%20me eting%20those%20goals%20successfully

- Gizer, I. R., Ficks, C., & Waldman, I. D. 2009. Candidate gene studies of ADHD: A meta-analytic review. *Human Genetics* 126(1): 51-90.

- Hallowell EM & Ratey JJ. 2021. *ADHD 2.0.* Sheldon Press, London.

- Holton KF & Nigg JT. 2020. The Association of Lifestyle Factors and ADHD in Children. *J Atten Disord.* 24(11): 1511-1520

- Huberman Lab. 2022. *Adderall, stimulants & modafinil for ADHD: Short- & long-term effects.* Huberman Lab podcast [Video]. YouTube.

https://www.youtube.com/watch?v=sxgCC4H1dl8

- Oades, R. 2007. Role of the serotonin system in ADHD: treatment implications. *Expert Rev Neurother.* 7(10):1357-74.

- Peterson, B. S., Trampush, J., Maglione, M., Bolshakova, M., Rozelle, M., & O'Neill, S. 2024. Treatments for ADHD in Children and Adolescents: A Systematic Review. *Pediatrics* 153(4): e2024065787. https://publications.aap.org/pediatrics/article/153/4/e2024065787/1 96922/Treatments-for-ADHD-in-Children-and-Adolescents-A

- Robbins, T. W., & Arnsten, A. F. T. 2009. The Neuropsychopharmacology of Fronto-Executive Function: Monoaminergic Modulation. *Annual Review of Neuroscience* 32(1): 267-287.

- Turic, D., Swanson, J. & Sonuga-Barke, E. 2010. DRD4 and DAT1 in ADHD: Functional neurobiology to pharmacogenetics. *Pharmgenomics Pers Med.* 3: 61-78.

- Wolraich, M. L., Feurer, I. D., Hannah, J. N., Baumgaertel, A., & Pinnock, T. Y. 1998. Examination of DSM-IV criteria for attention deficit/hyperactivity disorder in a county-wide sample. *Journal of Developmental & Behavioral Pediatrics* 19(3): 162-168.

- Yang, L., Liu, J., Sui, G., Chen, Y., & Guo, Y. 2017. Inflammation in attention-deficit/hyperactivity disorder (ADHD): A systematic review and meta-analysis of 39 studies. *Frontiers in Psychiatry* 8, Article 228. https://www.frontiersin.org/journals/psychiatry/articles/10.3389/fpsyt.2017.00228/full

www.ingramcontent.com/pod-product-compliance
Lightning Source LLC
Chambersburg PA
CBHW062049270326
41931CB00013B/2998

* 9 7 8 0 9 8 6 6 3 6 5 5 4 *